Tuina Therapy

Written by   Wang Daoquan

Translated by   Yan Menghui

                   Zhang Fan

Shandong Science and Technology Press

First Edition 1996

ISBN 7—5331—1839—1

Tuina Therapy

Written by	Wang Daoquan
Translated by	Yan Menghui
	Zhang Fan
Editor in charge	Li Yu

Published by Shandong Science and Technology Press

16 Yuhan Road, Jinan, China 250002

Printed by Shandong Dezhou Xinhua Printing House

Distributed by China International Book Trading Corporation

35 Chegongzhuang Xilu, Beijing 100044, China

P. O. Box 399, Beijing, China

Printed in the People's Republic of China

PREFACE

This book is one volumn of *The Series of Traditional Chinese Medicine for Foreign Readers*.

Tuina, also known as Chinese Massage, is one of the traditional Chinese medical therapies. As an invaluable legacy of the Chinese medicines, it has been well received among people in general, for its simple manipulation, easy learning, striking curative effects, safty, etc.

This book is composed of three parts. Part one issustuates sixty-five Tuina manoeuvres commonly used in clinical practice. Part two introduces seventy-three locales and points frequently operated on. Part three expounds forty-four common diseases and their corresponding treatments. In addition, 215 diagrams and 35 typical cases are included to facilitate a better understanding of Tuina therapy.

The book, for its richness in content, pithiness in compiling style and succinctness in language, may be used as a reference for practitioners on clinical practice, reseachers in medical study, or teachers and students in pedagogical training. Moreover, it is also applicable to households to prevent and cure various diseases.

CONTENTS

3

MANIPULATIONS
FOR ADULTS

Individual Manipulations

1. Pressing

Manipulation: Attach the thumb (Fig. 1) or overlapped palms (Fig. 2) tightly to the patient's body surface, and press on the affected locale with force. Pressing with the Thumb is suitable for various parts of the body and Pressing with the Overla-

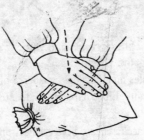

Fig. 1 Pressing with the Thumb

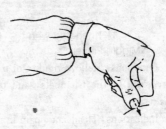

Fig. 2 Pressing with the Overlapped Palms

1

pped Palms for the lumbar region or lower limbs. The pressing strength should be gradually increased. It is contraindicated to exert brutal actions on the patient. Perform the operation for 0. 5 — 1 minute.

Functions: Relax muscles, promote Blood circulation to stop pain, and dredge the obstructed Channels.

Indications: Headache, epigastralgia, lumbago, backache, soreness, pain and numbness of the limbs, etc.

2. Kneading with the Finger

Manipulation: Attach the tip or belly of the middle finger (Fig. 3) or the thumb (see Fig. 4) tightly to a selected area of the patient's body surface, and knead it clockwise or anticlockwise with the finger moving revolvingly and the wrist and metacarpophalangeal joints as the driving source. Repeat the actions for 30—50 times.

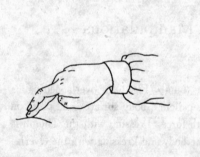 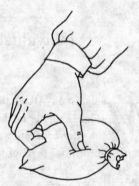

Fig. 3 Kneading with the   Fig. 4 Kneading with
        Middle Finger   the Thumb

Functions: Relieve rigidity of muscles and Tendons, disperse obstruction in the Channels, and promote Blood circulation to stop pain.

Indications: Headache, pain in the neck, chest, back, waist, and abdomen, soreness and numbness of the limbs.

3. Kneading with the Thenar Eminence

Manipulation: Apply strength through the thenar eminence, and

2

knead a selected part of the
patient's body surface circularly
(Fig. 5). It is recommended
that the wrist joint be relaxed
and the forearm sway actively
with the elbow as a propelling
point. Perform the actions for
3—5 minutes.

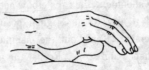

Fig. 5 Kneading with
Thenar Eminence

Functions: Smooth Qi and Blood circulation, remove Blood Stasis, promote subsidence of swelling, alleviate pain, relieve the stagnated and improve digestion.

Indications: Headache, dizziness, gastrointestinal disorders like
epigastralgia and constipation, and also for redness, swelling, and
pain caused by trauma.

4. Kneading with the Palm Base

Manipulation: Attach the palm base closely to a diseased part and
move circularly together with the wrist and forearm (Fig. 6). During the operation, the wrist joint should be relaxed and move round
and round with the elbow as its driving point. The kneading
strength should be gradually increased, from mild to heavy. This
manoeuvre is often used on the waist, back and limbs. Carry out the
performance for 3—5 minutes.

Functions: Relax muscles and
Tendons, promote Blood circula-
tion, dredge the Channels and
Collaterals to stop pain.

Indications: Backache, omalgia, lumbago, soreness, pain
and numbness of the limbs, etc.

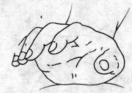

Fig. 6 Kneading with
the Palm Base

5. Rolling

Manipulation: Attach the ulnar side of your hand or the knuckles
of the middle, ring and little fingers to a certain area, and roll the
hand circularly with flexion and extension of the wrist joint and the
revolving of the forearm (Fig. 7—10). During the operation, lower

3

your shoulders, flex the elbow and wrist joint slightly, and keep the hand tightly to its original position with no dragging or sliding movement. Carry out the manipulation with appropriate pressure, frequency and scope. Repeat the method 120—160 times.

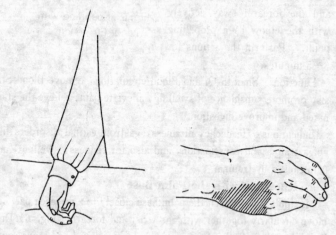

Fig. 7　Posture in Rolling　　Fig. 8　Attaching Part of the
　　　　　　　　　　　　　　　　　　 Hand in Rolling

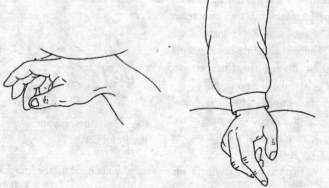

Fig. 9　Flexing the Wrist and　　Fig. 10　Extending the Wrist and
Everting the Forearm　　　　　　　　Inverting the Forearm

Functions: Relax muscles and Tendons, promote Blood circula-

4

tion to stop pain, relieve rigidity of joints, remit muscular and ligamentous spasm and strengthen their mobility, get rid of fatigue and tiredness.

Indications: Rheumatic pain and numbness in the shoulder, back, waist, buttocks and limbs, acroparalysis, dyskinesia, etc.

6. Grasping

Manipulation: Apply strength to a selected area through the five digital tips of one hand or both hands. Grasp the area by lifting and pinching the skin with the fingers dexterously and rhythmically. The strength applied should be increased step by step. It is contraindictive to exert a sudden and brutal force lest the skin be scratched. This method is often used to treat diseases of the neck (see Fig. 11), shoulder (Fig. 12) and the four limbs. Perform it 3—5 minutes each time.

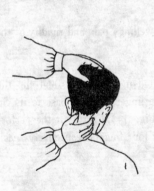 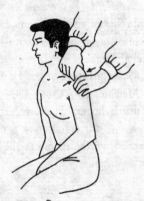

Fig. 11 Grasping the Neck   Fig. 12 Grasping the Shoulder

Functions: Expel Pathogenic Wind and Cold, promote the flow of Qi and Blood, relieve muscular and joint rigidity, disperse obstruction in the Channels, induce rescucitation and stop pain.

Indications: Common Cold, stiffness and pain in the neck, backache, soreness and pain of the limb joints.

7. Twisting

Manipulation: Form pincers with the tips of the thumb and index finger, hold and twist the affected finger nimbly, dexterously, pow-

5

erfully and rhythmically (Fig. 13). Avoid heavy and stagnant actions in manipulation. It is often used in the treatment of diseases of the finger or toe. Repeat the manoeuvre 3—5 minutes.

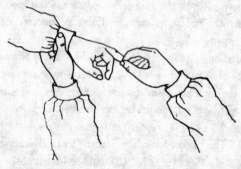

Fig. 13 Twisting

Functions: Relax muscles and Tendons, ease Blood circulation, and relieve rigidity of joints.

Indications: Sprain, contusion, swelling, pain and rigidity of the digital joints.

8. Regulating

Manipulation: Crook the index and middle fingers and clip the patient's finger. Then, regulate the finger from its base to its tip with even force and quick action (Fig. 14). Carry out the performance from the thumb to the other four fingers respectively, each for 2—5 times.

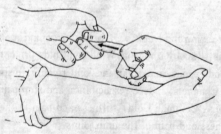

Fig. 14 Regulating

Functions: Clear the Channels and Collaterals, promote the flow of Qi, and ease Blood circulation.

Indications: Digital pain and numbness due to trauma, peripheral neuritis, etc.

9. Dotting with the Flexed Finger

Manipulation: Press your flexed thumb (Fig. 15) or flexed index finger (Fig. 16) firmly onto the patient's body surface. Induce Qi into the pressing point and increase the pressing strength gradually until the patient perceives a sensation of soreness, numbness, distention, pain and heaviness radiating around the locale, which is called the arrival of Qi.

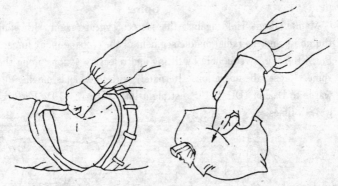

Fig. 15 Dotting with the   Fig. 16 Dotting with the Flexed
Flexed Thumb   Index Finger

Functions: Dredge the obstructed, activate Blood circulation to stop pain, and regulate functions of Zang and Fu organs.

Indications: Spasmodic pain in the epigastric regions, pain in the loins and legs, stiff-neck, etc.

10. Dotting with the Middle Finger

Manipulation: Support the middle segment of the middle finger with bellies of the thumb and index finger. Concentrate Qi into the middle finger. Press the fingertip firmly onto the selected point (Fig. 17). During operation, the forearm should be slightly elevated, the elbow flexed, the wrist bent downwards. Perform the maneouvre 1—3 times for each point.

Functions: Relieve muscular rigidity, disperse obstruction in the Channels, promote the flow of Qi and Blood, regulate the functions

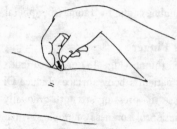

Fig. 17 Dotting with the
Middle Finger

of Zang and Fu, disperse
Pathogenic Cold and assuage
pain.

Indications: Hemiplegia, rigidity and numbness of joints,
arthralgia due to Wind-Cold-
Dampness, and Flaccidity Syndrome.

11. Pinching along the Spine

Manipulation: Hold against the sacrococcygeal region with your
thumb tip and the radial middle segment of the crooked index finger.
Pinch the skin strenuously by lifting and releasing actions along the
spine. Repeat the operations alternately with two hands moving upwards to Dazhui (DU 14) in a straight line (Fig. 18—19). Perform
it 3—5 times.

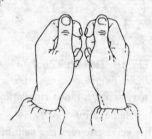 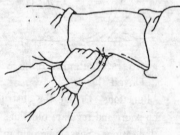

Fig. 18 Pinching along the   Fig. 19 Pinching along the
Spine(1):Front View   Spine (2):Side View

Functions: Clear the Channels and Collaterals, regulate Qi and
Blood, Yin and Yang, Zang and Fu, and reinforce Vital Qi.

Indications: Insomnia, neurosism, gastrointestinal diseases, irregular menstruation, etc.

12. Plucking

Manipulation: Attach the thumb tip or the triangular plane of
your flexed elbow to a diseased part or point. Press and move the
selected locale with the thumb to and fro with force (Fig. 20). The

8

strength applied should be gradually increased, from mild to heavy. Do it 3—5 times.

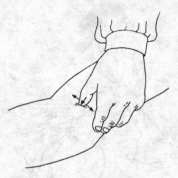

Fig. 20 Plucking

Functions: Promote the circulation of Qi and Blood, detach adhesion, and relieve convulsion and pain.

Indications: Tennis elbow, syndrome of M. piriformis, chronic lumbar muscle strain, etc.

13. Scraping

Manipulation: The patient lies supine or prone. The practitioner takes an instrument like a cup or spoon of smooth edges and puts it on such locale as either side of the spine, the neck, hyponchondrium, abdomen, cubital fossa or popliteal fossa, etc. Then, scrape the part up and down until there appears congestion or purplish red eccymosis on the portion operated on (Fig. 21). Some media may be used in operation lest the skin be injured.

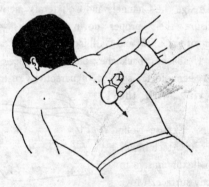

Fig. 21 Scraping

Functions: Purge Pathogenic Heat from Blood, activate Blood flow, send down the upward adverse flow of Qi, arrest vomiting, promote digestion, and resolve masses.

Indications: Fever due to exopathy, sunstroke, vomiting, diarrhea, and oppressed feeling in the chest.

14. Revolving with the Flexed Elbow

Manipulation: Attach the triangular plane of the flexed elbow closely to a selected spot, then move it on the spot revolvingly again and again with high frequency (Fig. 22). The revolving force should be soft and mild but deepening and penetrating. This manoeuvre is commonly applied to such points as Huantiao (G 30), Chengfu (B 50), and Yinmen (B 51), which contain corpulent muscles. It is better to repeat the therapy for 3—5 minutes until the patient gets a local warm sensation.

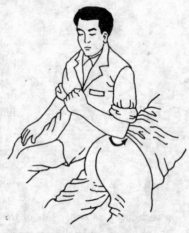

Fig. 22 Revolving with the Flexed Elbow

Functions: Dredge the Channels and Collaterals, activate Qi and Blood and ensure their proper downward flow, clear away Pathogenic Heat of the Liver and Gallbladder.

Indications: Headache, backache, pain in the neck and lower limbs, lumbago, hemiplegia, sciatica, hyperactivity of Liver Yang.

15. Revolving with the Forearm

Manipulation: Expose your forearm and flex it, attach its ulnar aspect with flexor muscle to the patient's body surface. Move the forearm on the locale revolvingly with a mild, soft, but deepening and penetrating force (Fig. 23).

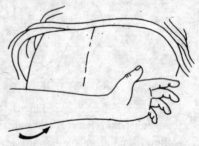

Fig. 23 Revolving with the Forearm

Functions: Relax muscles and Tendons, promote Blood circulation, remove muscular and ligamental spasm and convulsion.

Indications: Pain, numbness, and dysfunction of the neck, shoulder waist and limbs.

16. Suppressing with the Flexed Elbow

Manipulation: Flex the elbow, with palm facing chest. Press down a selected area powerfully with the elbow tip persistently or intermittently, with or without the help of the other hand (Fig. 24). The suppressing strength should be increased gradually from mild to heavy. The operation may last 1—3 minutes.

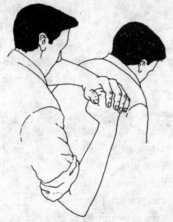

Fig. 24   Suppressing with the Flexed Elbow

Functions: Remove Pathogenic Wind and Cold, promote the flow of Qi and Blood, remove obstruction in the Channels and Collaterals, relieve convulsion and stop pain.

Indications: Rheumatic Arthralgia Syndrome, distending pain in the loins and back, sciatica, contracture of the limbs, etc.

17. Rubbing with Both Palms

Manipulation: Apply opposite strength through both entire palms, and rub a selected part inwards and outwards from above with high frequency (Fig. 25). Perform it briskly, dexterously, symmetrically and rhythmically. This manoeuvre is often used on the four limbs at the end of a treatment. Perform it 1—2 times on each locale.

Functions: Relieve rigidity of muscles and Tendons, clear and activate the Channels and Collaterals, and regulate the flow of Qi and Blood.

Indications: Distension, pain, and malaise in the limbs and hypochondriac regions.

18. Rubbing with Both Thenar Eminences

Manipulation: Ask the patient to raise his (her) hand, with the dorsum facing the practitioner. Hold his (her) ring and little fingers

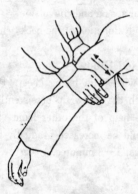

Fig. 25 Rubbing with Both Palms

with one hand and the thumb and index fingers with the other. Induce strength into the hand dorsum with the two palms and rub it alternatively in a brisk, flexible and skillful way (Fig. 26). Repeat the operation 10 — 20 times until a warm sensation is perceived by the patient.

Functions: Relax muscles and

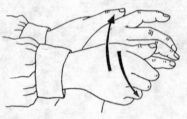

Fig. 26 Rubbing with Both Thenar Eminences

Tendons, ease Blood circulation, disperse obstruction in the Channels and Collaterals to alleviate pain.

Indications: Digital numbness, grasping debility, cold and pain sensation in the extremities, contracture and spasm of muscles and Tendons.

19. Round-rubbing

Manipulation: Induce strength into a selected area and rub it with the entire palm (Fig. 27) or the fingers (the index, middle, and ring) (Fig. 28) circularly and persistently. In doing so, relax the wrist joint and branch the fingers off naturally. Use even force and rhythmical movement. This manoeuvre is often applied to the abdomen. Carry it out for 3—5 minutes on the part operated on.

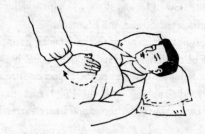

Fig. 27   Round-rubbing with the Palm

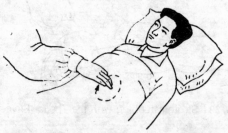

Fig. 28   Round-rubbing with the Fingers

Functions: Relieve retention of stagnated food, regulate the Middle Jiao and Qi, normalize enterogastric functions, relax muscles and Tendons, and smooth Blood circulation.

Indications: Distension, tightness and pain in the epigastrium, abdomen, chest, or hypochondrium, indigestion, constipation, diarrhea, redness, swelling and pain caused by trauma.

20. Straight-rubbing (Burning)

Manipulation: Rub in a straight line an affected portion with the thenar eminence of the right hand (Fig. 29), or its palm (Fig. 30), or its polythenar eminences (Fig. 31). Perform the operation with even, steady, persistent and rhythmical force and natural respiration. The friction pressure should be appropriate, and the scope be large. The part to be operated on should be exposed and a dress-insulating operation is not desirable. Some medium like massage oil

- 13

may be used lest the skin be injured. Repeat it 100—200 times until there appears a burning sensation on the locale.

Functions: Warm and clear the Channels, expel Wind, dissipate Cold, promote the flow of Qi and Blood, subdue swelling to assuage pain, and strengthen the Spleen and Stomach.

Indications: Straight-rubbing with the Thenar Eminence is suitable for diseases of the limbs, chest, abdomen, and back; Straight-rubbing with the Palm for diseases in the hypochondriac and abdominal regions; Straight-rubbing with the Polythenar Eminences for disorders in the back, waist, buttocks and lower extremities.

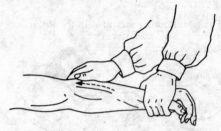

Fig. 29   Straight-rubbing with the Thenar Eminence

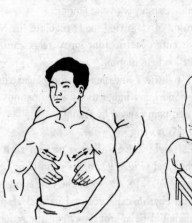

Fig. 30   Straight-rubbing
with the Palm

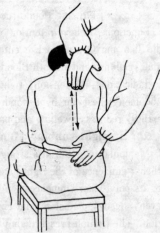

Fig. 31   Straight-rubbing with
the Polythenar Eminences

14

21. Pushing

Manipulation: Apply strength to a diseased portion through the thumb belly (Fig. 32), or the palm (Fig. 33), or the triangular plane of the flexed elbow (Fig. 34). Manipulate by forward pushing slowly and steadily. Do pushing 3—5 times on the locale.

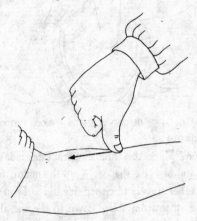

Fig. 32 Pushing with the Tumb

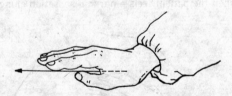

Fig. 33 Pushing with the Palm

Functions: Relax muscles and Tendons, promote Blood circulation, and disperse obstruction in the Channels and Collaterals.

Indications: Pushing with the Thumb is suitable for diseases in the head, neck, and upper extremities; Pushing with the Palm for diseases in the lower limbs, waist and back; Pushing with the Flexed Elbow for soreness and pain in the lumbar and back regions.

15

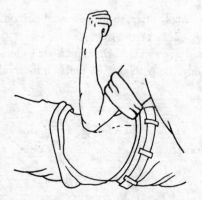

Fig. 34   Pushing with the Flexed Elbow

22. Scratching

Manipulation: Make the three fingers (the index, middle, and ring) of one hand be hook-shaped. Keep the middle finger closely to the spine and other fingers to either side of it. Then scratch powerfully along the spine from above down to the sacral portion (Fig. 35). This manoeuvre should be implemented with a high frequency. Avoid injuries of the skin during operation. Good results will be obtained when the patient feels a burning sensation along the spine.

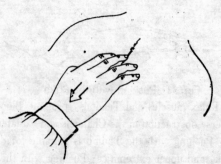

Fig. 35   Scratching

Functions: Get rid of muscular tightness, treat Exterior Syndrome, warm up the Middle Jiao, smooth Qi-Blood circulation, dredge the obstructed and remove the stagnated, strengthen the

16

body resistance and clear away the exogenous pathogens.

Indications: Common cold caused by Pathogenic Wind and Cold, soreness and pain in the back and waist, aversion to chills, cold limbs, lassitude, listlessness, anorexia, etc.

23. Wiping

Manipulation: Apply strength to a diseased part through the belly of a thumb or bellies of both thumbs. Wipe the area with flexing and extending of the thumb or thumbs to and fro repeatedly (Fig. 36). The wiping strength should be mild but not floating, heavy but not stagnant. Repeat the actions 30—50 times.

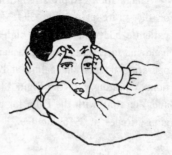

Fig. 36 Wiping

Functions: Induce resuscitation, refresh the mind, and promote acuity of vision.

Indications: Dizziness, headache, stiffness and pain in the neck and nape.

24. Shaking

Manipulation: Hold the farther end of the patient's lower or upper limb with both hands, shake it up and down persistently and powerfully with a high frequency (Fig. 37). The manipulation and scope should be gradually increased, from small to large. Perform the operations 1 or 2 times. Clinically, it is often used together with Rubbing with Both Palms as an end during a course of Tuina therapy.

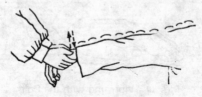

Fig. 37 Shaking

Functions: Relax muscles and Tendons, purge obstruction in the Channels and Collaterals, regulate the flow of Qi and Blood.

Indications: Soreness, pain and numbness of the limbs, etc.

25. Vibrating

Manipulation: Apply strength through the finger tips (Fig. 38) or the entire palm (Fig 39). Vibrate on a certain part of the patient's body surface with high frequency and static force of the hand and forearm. During the manipulation, be concentrated on the operating fingers and palm, and manipulate with natural respiration. Vibrating with the Digital Tips is suitable for various points, and Vibrating with the Palm for the abdominal and lumbosacral regions. Repeat it 2—5 minutes.

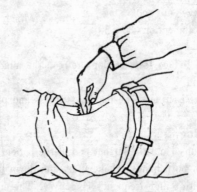

Fig. 38   Vibrating with the Fingers

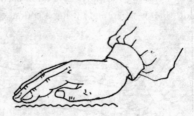

Fig. 39   Vibrating with the Palm

Functions: Dredge the Channels, remove Blood Stasis, promote digestion and relieve flatulence, normalize the functions of the gastrointestines, middle Jiao, and the flow of Qi.

Indications: Headache, dizziness, insomnia, lumbago, epigastralgia, abdominal pain and distention, diarrhea, etc.

26. Knocking

Manipulation: According to the gestures, Knocking manoeuvre is commonly divided into the following types: Knocking with the Fist, often used on the waist and back (Fig. 40); Knocking with the Palm Base, commonly applied to the buttocks or lower extremities (Fig. 41); Knocking with the Ulnar Polythenar Eminences, mostly used on the waist and lower extremities (Fig. 42), and Knocking with the Digital Tips, used on the head (Fig. 43). All the actions should be gentle, quick, skillful and rhythmical. Avoid dragging movement. The operation may be repeated 3—5 times on each locale.

Functions: Relax muscles and Tendons, expel obstruction in the Channels and Collaterals, regulate the flow of Qi and Blood.

Indications: Arthralgia caused by Wind-Cold-Dampness, local dysesthesia, numbness, soreness and pain in the waist, back, and lower limbs, myospasm, headache, hemiplegia, etc.

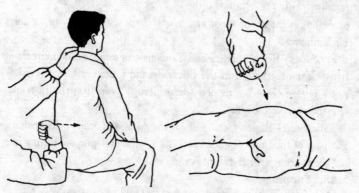

Fig. 40　Knocking with
the Fist

Fig. 41　Knocking with the
Palm Base

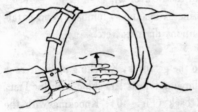

Fig. 42　Knocking with the Ulnar Polythnar Eminences

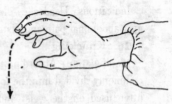

Fig. 43　Knocking with the Fingers

27. Chopping with the Joined Palms

Manipulation: Join the palms of both hands together, with the fingers outstretched naturally. Apply strength to a selected locale by knocking through the ulnar side of the joined hands (Fig. 44). Chopping sound can be heard in the operation. The manoeuvre should be performed rapidly, with the elbow as the propelling point of the wrist and hands. Repeat the performance for 1—3 minutes.

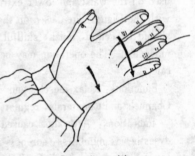

Fig. 44　Chopping with the Joined Palms

Functions: Relax muscles and Tendons to promote Blood circulation, clear obstruction in the Channels and Collaterals to alleviate pain, relieve chest oppression, stop hiccup, normalize the flow of Qi, and resolve phlegm.

Indications: Rigidity and pain in the back and waist, distension and pain of the limbs, general asthenia, full and depressed feeling in the chest, cough with dyspnea, etc.

28. Tapping

Manipulation: Crook the five fingers of one hand slightly to form a void palm. Then tap a diseased area steadily and rhythmically for 3 —5 times (Fig. 45).

20

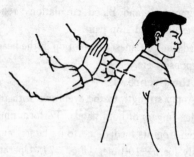

Fig. 45 Tapping

Functions: Relieve stiff muscles and Tendons, disperse obstruction in the Channels and Collaterals, promote Qi and Blood circulation, and it can also excite muscles.

Indications: Rheumatic pain in the shoulder, back, waist, buttocks andlower limbs, local dysesthesia, numbness, muscular spasm, chronic lumbar muscle strain, etc.

29. Pushing the Forehead Divergently

Manipulation: Induce strength to the patient's forehead through the bellies of both thumbs. Push the patient's forehead divergently from Yintang (Ex-HN) to the lateral hairlines, while passing the anterior hairlines (Fig. 46). The strength applied should be mild and soft. Manipulate it 30-50 times.

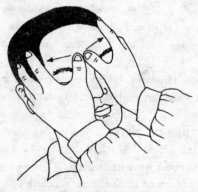

Fig. 46 Pushing the Forehead Divergently

Functions: Promote Qi and Blood circulation, relieve mental strain, improve eyesight, and stop pain.

Indications: Headache, dizziness, distention in the head, insomnia, dreaminess, hypopsia, etc.

30. Pinching the Eyebrows

Manipulation: Apply strength to the eyebrows with the bellies of the thumb and index fingers of both hands. Perform pinching along the superciliary arch from its medial end to its lateral nimbly, flexibly and dexterously for 5—10 times (Fig. 47). Operate on either eyebrow for 5—10 times.

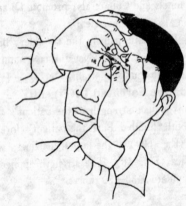

Fig. 47   Pinching the Eyebrows

Functions: Disperse Pathogenic Wind, relieve Exterior Syndrome, clear the mind and eyes, ease mental stress, and assuage headache.

Indications: Headache due to common cold, insomnia, dreaminess, dryness and foreign-body sensation in the eyes, fatigue of vision, myopia, etc.

31. Rotating the Neck

Manipulation: Hold the back of the patient's head with one hand, and his (her) lower jaw with the other. Turn the patient's head and neck round and round clockwise or anticlockwise repeatedly (Fig. 48). Increase the rotating force gradually according to limitation of

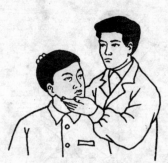

Fig. 48 Rotating the Neck

the physiological movement of the patient. Repeat the actions 3 — 5 times.

Functions: Clear the Channels and Collaterals in the neck, remove its rigidity and improve the motor functions of its joints.

Indications: Pain and rigidity in the neck region, stiff-neck, cervical spondylopathy, etc.

32. Pulling the Neck Semi-circularly

Manipulation: Support with one hand the back part of the patient's head, which is slightly bent forwards, and fix his (her) lower jaw with the other hand. Turn the patient's head sideward to its largest degree, then pull the head and neck suddenly and strenuously towards the opposite direction (Fig. 49). During the dirigation, the patient should incline anteriorly. Perform it once to the left and to the right respectively.

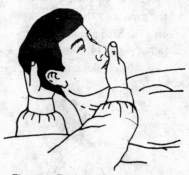

Fig. 49 Pulling the Neck Semi-circularly

Functions: Relax muscular rigidity, clear and activate the Channels and Collaterals, lubricate stiff joints, correct deformity of the neck.

Indications: Stiffneck, malposition of the minor articulations in the cervical vertebrae, etc..

33. Pulling up the Neck

Manipulation: Stand behind the patient who is sitting. Support and fix the back of the patient's head with both thumbs and his (her) lower jaw with both palm bases, while suppressing the patient's shoulders with both forearms. When all this is done, pull up the patient's neck with both hands (Fig. 50). If the patient is fat, carry out the manipulation on a therapeutic bed. Ask the patient to lie supinely and relax completely. Stand facing his (her) head, support his (her) lower jaw with one hand and the nape with the other, then drag the head and neck power-

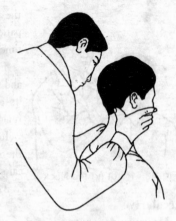

Fig. 50 Pulling up the Neck: the Sitting Posture

fully (Fig. 51). The strength applied should be increased step by step. Repeat the actions 1—2 minutes or 5—10 times.

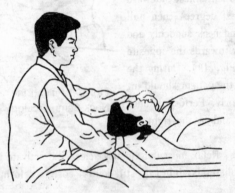

Fig. 51 Pulling up the Neck: the Lying Posture

Functions: Help to form cervical vertebral spaces, promote the wry neck to return to its original position, relax muscles and Tendons, relieve rigidity of joints, and detach articular adhesion.

Indications: Cervical spondylopathy, protrusion of the cervical intervertebral disc, dislocation of the cervical vertebrae, etc.

24

34. Lifting the Head and Neck

Manipulation: The patient sits on a lower stool, and the practitioner takes a semi-squatting posture. Fix the patient's lower jaw tightly with the left flexed arm, and his (her) occipital part with the right hand (Fig. 52). Then stand up slowly, while lifting the patient's head and neck upwards (Fig. 53). The downward tugging force of the patient's body will help to stretch his (her) cervical vertebrae. The lifting strength should be applied evenly and steadily and the lifting action may last 1—2 minutes.

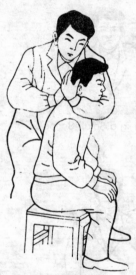 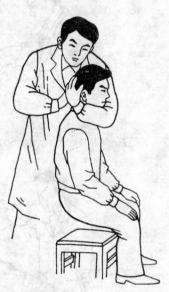

Fig. 52 Lifting the
Head and Neck (1)

Fig. 53 Lifting the
Head and Neck (2)

Functions: Relax muscles and Tendons, clear and activate the Channels and Collaterals, form definite intervertebral spaces, treat traumatic tissues and benefit reposition of prolapsed intervertebral disc.

Indications: Cervical spondylopathy, fissure of the vertebrae, protrusion of the cervical intervertebral disc, etc.

35. Rotating the Shoulder

25

Manipulation: The patient sits on a stool. Put one hand on his (her) shoulder and the other hand under his (her) elbow. Move the patient's shoulder round and round in a small scope (Fig. 54). Afterwards, hold his (her) wrist with one hand and his (her) shoulder with the other hand, and carry out rotation of the shoulder in a large scope and increasing force (Fig. 55—57). Perform it clockwise or anticlockwise 3—5 times to an appropriate extent.

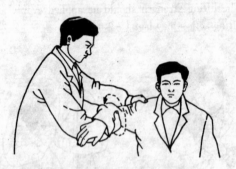

Fig. 54   Rotating the Shoulder in a Small Scope

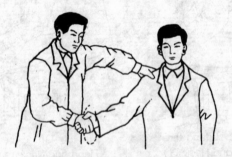

Fig. 55   Rotating the Shoulder in a Large Scope (1)

Functions: Lubricate stiff joints, scatter articular adhesion, and promote motor functions of the joint.

Indications: Scapulohumeral periarthritis, soreness and pain in the shoulder and arm, dysfunction of the shoulder joint.

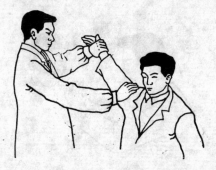

Fig. 56　Rotating the Shoulder in a Large Scope （2）

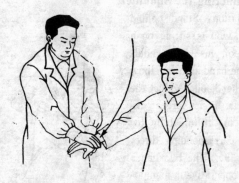

Fig. 57　Rotating the Shoulder in a Large Scope （3）

36. Abducting the Shoulder

Manipulation: The patient sits on a stool. The practitioner takes a posture of semi-squatting. Stand up slowly while suppressing the patient's shoulder with the crossed hands. When it is extended to its largest degree, abduct the patient's shoulder joint with a sudden and powerful strength (Fig. 58). The operating scope should be gradually enlarged. The patient who suffers from hypertension or coronary heart disease should adopt it cautiously.

Functions: Separate adhesion, lubricate stiff joints, help to restore the functions of the shoulder.

Indications: Omalgia, scapulohumeral periarthritis, disturbance in shoulder movements.

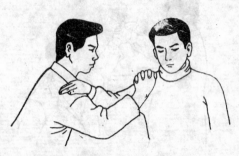

Fig. 58　Abducting the Shoulder

37. Adducting the Shoulder

Manipulation: Stand behind the patient who is sitting on a stool. Support his (her) shoulder with one hand and the elbow with the other hand. Adduct the shoulder joint to its largest extent, then tug it forcefully towards the corresponding direction (Fig. 59). The two hands should be cooperative in manipulation, and the tugging actions be brisk and rapid. Perform it in the proper physiological scope for 1—2 times.

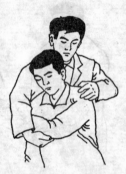

Fig. 59　Adducting the Shoulder

Functions: Lubricate stiff joints and scatter adhesion.

Indications: Scapulohumeral periarthritis, disturbance of shoulder activities, etc.

38. Extending and Flexing the Shoulder

Manipulation: The patient sits on a stool. Hold his (her) wrist with one hand and support the shoulder with the other hand. Extend the patient's arm forward to its largest extent, then pull it with more strength in the same direction. Afterwards, flex the patient's

28

arm backward and exert more strength in the corresponding direction (Fig. 60−61). The actions should be briskly and rapidly carried out. Manipulate it 1 or 2 times within the appropriate physiological scope.

Functions: The same as mentioned in Abducting the Shoulder.

Indications: Scapulohumeral periarthritis, disturbance in shoulder movements, etc.

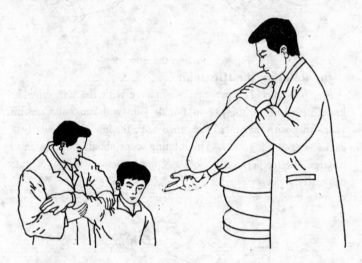

Fig. 60　Extending the　　Fig. 61　Flexing the Shoulder
Shoulder Forwards　　　　Backwards

39. Pulling the Shoulder

Manipulation: Hold the wrist or elbow of the patient with both hands, pull the arm with increasing strength to stretch the shoulder joint. Bid the patient to sit steadily with his (her) body inclining to the opposite direction (or fix the body by an assistant) (Fig. 62). The strength applied should be even and persistent. Repeat the actions for 0.5−1 minute.

Functions: Relax muscles and Tendons, facilitate Blood circulation, treat traumatic tissues, lubricate joints and help restore to their normal functions.

Indications: Damaged muscles and bones in the shoulder region,

29

dysfunction caused by periarthritis of shoulder at its anaphase.

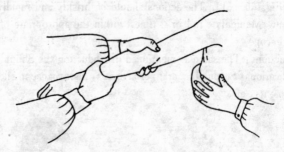

Fig. 62   Pulling the Shoulder

40. Rotating the Hip Joint

Manipulation: The patient lies supinely with the hip joint and knees flexed. Hold the patient's ankle joint with one hand and his (her) knee with the other hand, then move the hip joint circularly again and again (Fig. 63). The rotating scope should be from small to large. Better perform it clockwise and anticlockwise 3—5 times respectively.

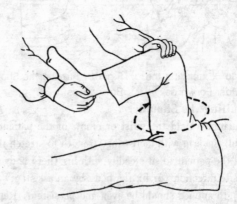

Fig. 63   Rotating the Hip Joint

Functions: Relax muscles and Tendons to alleviate arthralgia, activate Blood circulation, clear the Channels and Collaterals, and lubricate joints.

Indications: Injuries of the soft tissues in the hip region,

30

coxarthritis, sacro-iliilis, dysfunction of the hip joint, etc.

41. Extending the Chest

Manipulation: Ask the patient to sit with his (her) two hands clasped on the nape. Stand behind the patient, support his (her) back with one knee, then extend the patient's chest by pulling the patient's arms with the two hands powerfully (Fig. 64). The patient should relax his (her) body completely with deep inspiration during the manipulation. The hugging should be finished skillfully in an instant. Repeat it 1—2 times.

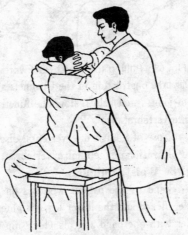

Fig. 64   Extending the CHest

Functions: Relax muscles and Tendons, clear the Channels and Collaterals, treat injured soft tissues and help restore dislocated bones.

Indications: Trauma in the hypochondriac region, disturbance of activities and pain of the shoulder joint, disorders of the costovertebral articulations, depressed feeling and stabbing pain in the chest.

42. Pulling the Waist Backward

Manipulation: Ask the patient to lie prone with his (her)lower limbs joined together. Pull the patient's legs upward with one hand while pressing his (her) lumbar region downward with the other. When the patient's waist is bent backwards to its largest degree, exert greater traction strength with the two hands in opposite directions (Fig. 65). The manipulation scope should be gradually enlarged in accordance with limitation of the patient's physiological movement. Repeat it 2—5 times.

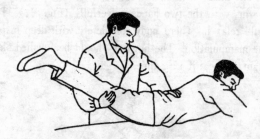

Fig. 65   Pulling the Waist Backward

Functions: Disperse obstruction in the Channels and Collaterals, relieve rigidity of joints, and help restore the functions of the prolapsed lumbar intervertebral disc .

Indications: Prolapse of lumbar intervertebral disc, sprain in the waist, backward protrusion of the lumbar vertebrae, etc.

43. Pulling the Waist Obliquely

Manipulation: Stand by the patient who lies on his (her) side with the upper leg flexed and the lower leg straightened. Press the patient's shoulder with one hand and his (her) hip with the other hand. Pull the two parts simultaneously with the two hands in opposite directions so as to stretch the lumbar region (Fig. 66). The successful signal is a crack which can be heard by the practitioner. Carry it out first on the diseased side, then on the healthy side, once respectively.

Functions: Extend the spinal vertebrae, relax their adjacent muscles and Tendons, activate the Channels and Collaterals, lubricate stiff joints, separate adhesion, and benefit reposition of dislocated joints.

Indications: Prolapse of intervertebral disc, hypertrophic inflammation and synovial incarceration of minor articulations in lumbar vertebrae, muscular strain in the lumbar region.

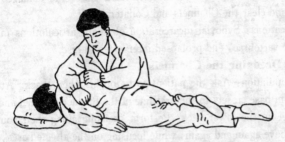

Fig. 66 Pulling the Waist Obliquely

44. Pulling the Waist Semi-circularly

Manipulation: Ask an assistant to stabilize the lower limbs and pelvis of the patient who is sitting. Stand behind the patient, support his (her) diseased side of the waist with one hand, and his (her) neck with the other hand which passes through his (her) armpit. Pull the patient's waist towards the diseased side to its greatest degree, then exert more strength to tug it in the same direction (Fig. 67 — 68). At this moment, a crack sound may be heard, which indicates the lumbar vertebra is repositioned. Then, carry out the manipulation on the healthy side in the same way. All the actions should be done in harmonious coordination. Do it once or twice on either side .

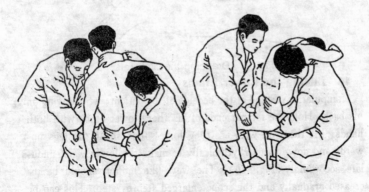

Fig. 67 Pulling the
Waist Semi-circularly (1)

Fig. 68 Pulling the
Waist Semi-circularly (2)

Functions: Help restore the dislocated joints and damaged tissues, and clear the Channels and Collaterals.

Indications: Synovial incarceration of minor articulations in the lumbar vertebrae, and prolapsed intervertebral disc.

45. Dredging the Channels

Manipulation: Ask the patient to lie on his (her) back. Attach the palm base closely to the first line of the Bladder Channel and Du Channel on the lower back. Perform kneading along their courses from above again and again, while focusing on the affected area, until a warm sensation is perceived by the patient (Fig. 69). The strength applied should be mild first, then heavy, then mild again. Repeat the Tuina manoeuvre 3—5 minutes.

Functions: Promote Blood circulation, relieve convulsion and stop pain, and eliminate muscular overfatigue in the waist and back.

Indications: Soreness, pain, stiffness of the waist and back, lumbar muscle strain, retrograde inflammation in the lumbar vertebrae, prolapse of the intervertebral disc.

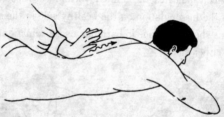

Fig. 69   Dredging the Channels

46. Lifting the Lower Limbs

Manipulation: Stand at the bedside of the patient, who is lying on his back. Hold the farther ends of his (her) lower limbs with both hands, lift them up with a strong force, then shake the legs upwards and downwards rhythmically to make the lower waist undulate accordingly (Fig. 70). The wave-like motion should be increased gradually and the scope enlarged step by step. This can be performed 3—5 times successively.

34

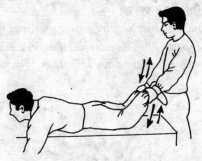

Fig. 70   Lifting the Lower Limbs

Functions: Relax muscles and Tendons, clear and activate the Channels and Collaterals, lubricate stiff joints, and detach adhesion.

Indications: Prolapse of intervertebral disc, dysfunction of minor articulations in the lumbar vertebrae.

47. Pulling the Wrist

Manipulation: Hold the lower part of the patient's forearm with one hand and his (her) hand with the other hand. Pull the wrist with the two hands in opposite directions (Fig. 71). Perform the operation with a steady and increasing force for 0.5—1 minute .

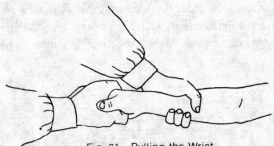

Fig. 71   Pulling the Wrist

Functions: Relax muscles and Tendons, clear and activate the Channels and Collaterals, help restore the malpositioned joint to its normal.

Indications: Sprain, contusion, dislocation and motor disturbance in the wrist joint .

48. Rotating the Wrist

Manipulation: Hold with both hands the wrist of the patient who is sitting on a chair. Rock it clockwise or anticlockwise in combination with pulling and dragging for 3—5 times (Fig. 72).

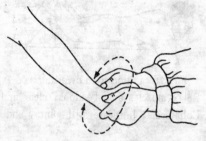

Fig. 72 Rotating the Wrist

Functions: Relax muscles and Tendons to smooth Blood circulation, lubricate stiff joints, and scatter adhesion in the wrist.

Indications: Sprain and contusion of the wrist joint, disturbance of activities in the wrist joint.

49. Pushing the Elbow

Manipulation: The patient sits on a chair. Hold his (her) wrist with one hand and attach the thenar eminence or palm of the other hand to the radial side of his (her) forearm, then do pushing on it to and fro in a straight line (Fig. 73). The pushing strength should be slowly and steadily applied. Repeat the actions 3—5 times on the locale.

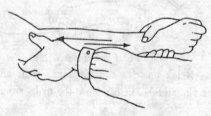

Fig. 73 Pushing the Elbow

Functions: Relax muscles and Tendons to promote Blood circulation, and promote muscular excitement.

Indications: External humeral epicondylitis, soreness, pain, and numbness in the forearm.

50. Pulling the Finger

Manipulation: Let the patient sit on a chair. Hold the part above the patient's wrist with one hand and clip one of his (her)fingers tightly with the other hand. Apply strength through pulling with both hands in opposite directions (Fig. 74). Manipulate with steady and even force, each finger for 0.5—1 minute.

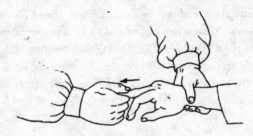

Fig. 74   Pulling the Finger

Functions: Help restore the injured tissues and malpositioned digital joints to their normal functions.

Indications: Sprain and contusion of the interphalangeal and metacarpophalangeal articulations, and disturbance in their flexion and extension.

51. Rotating the Finger

Manipulation: Seize the patient's wrist with one hand and pinch his (her) affected finger with the other hand. Rock the finger clockwise or anticlockwise 10—20 times (Fig. 75). The operating scope should be gradually increased. It is contraindicated to give a sudden and brutal action.

Functions: Relieve rigidity of the interphalangeal articulation, detach adhesion in it, and restore it to its original functions.

Indications: Interphalangeal sprain and contusion, dysfunction in digital flexion and extension, etc.

37

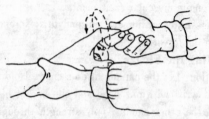

Fig. 75 Rotating the Finger

52. On-the-point Pressing

Manipulation: Crook the five fingers to form a void fist, and attach naturally the thumb tip to a certain spot. Sway the wrist to drive the thumb joint to flex and extend so as to produce downward force on the point (Fig. 76—79). During the operation, the practitioner should relax the wrist, droop the shoulder, and suspend the wrist with the elbow as its support. Use even force and appropriate pressure and frequency. Perform the manipulation 120—160 times per minute.

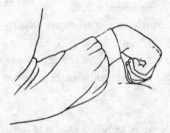
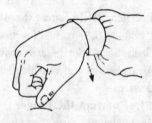

Fig. 76 On-the-point Pressing
(1):the Sitting Posture

Fig. 77 On-the-point Pressing
(2):Suspending the Wrist,
Forming a Void Fist,Attaching
the Thumb Naturally

Functions: Relax muscles and Tendons to promote Blood circulation, regulate Ying and Wei Levels, resolve Blood Stasis, remove stagnated food, and strengthen the Spleen and Stomach.

Indications: Headache, gastralgia, abdominal pain, soreness and pain of the limbs, etc.

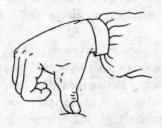 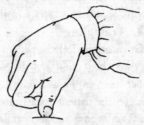

Fig. 78   On-the-point Pressing
(3):the Wrist Swinging Outward

Fig. 79   On-the-poin Pressing
(4):the Wrist Swinging Inward

53. Inserting

Manipulation: Stand behind the patient, who sits on a stool with the flexed arm on the lumbar region. Join the outstretched fingers together, insert the digital tips upwards along the lower medial margin of the patient's scapula to the depth $2-3$ cun between the scapula and the thoracic wall; at the same time, press the anterior part of the patient's shoulder with the other hand; afterwards, release the inserting hand slowly (see Fig. 80). The manipulation should be soft and mild but deepening and penetrating with increasing strength. Avoid sudden and brutal actions in inserting or releasing of the hand. It can be repeated $3-5$ times.

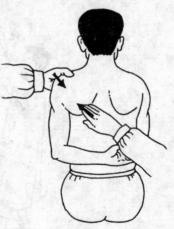

Fig. 80   Inserting

Functions: Elevate Spleen Qi, stretch muscles and Tendons, facilitate Blood circulation, regulate the Middle Jiao, relieve oppressed feeling in the chest.

Indications: Full and distending sensation in the abdomen (gas-

39

troptosia) especially after meal, emaciation, general debility, peri-arthritis of shoulder, strain of the supraspinous muscle, etc.

54. Trampling

Manipulation: Let the patient lie on his back. Put several pillows under his (her) chest and thighs to make the body higher and seize the bar fixed on the wall with both hands. Having finished all this, stamp on the patient's waist and spring on it in an appropriate extent. Don't move the feet while springing (Fig. 81). The patient should regulate his (her) breath in a correspondence with the trampling actions, exhaling while the heels fall down, and inhaling while the heels rise. The speed should be appropriate and the actions rhythmical. Repeat the manoeuvre 5—10 times. It is contraindicated to use this method on patients who are afflicted with senile osteoporosis, tuberculosis of spine, hypertension, or coronary heart disease.

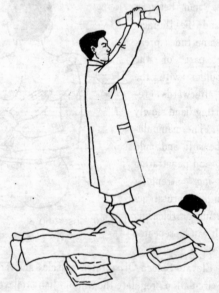

Fig. 81 Trampling

Functions: Restore and treat injured soft tissues, correct deformity, relieve rigidity of muscles and Tendons, clear and activate the

40

Channels and Collaterals.

Indications: Prolapse of intervertebral disc, kyphotic deformity, and lumbar muscle strain.

Integrated Manipulations

1. Nipping-grasping

Manipulation: Crook the five fingers of a hand and put them around an affected joint. Nip and grasp the point along the joint fissure skillfully and dexterously (Fig. 82). There is nipping in grasping and vice versa, there is grasping in nipping. The two manoeuvres should combined into an integrate unit. Good results will be obtained when the patient perceives a sore, distending, and warm sensation around the affected area.

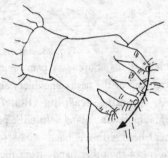

Fig. 82 Nipping grasping

Functions: Remove Pathogenic Wind and Cold, dredge the Channels, relax muscles and Tendons to promote Blood circulation, and lubricate stiff joints.

Indications: Pain, rigidity, and disturbance of activities in the shoulder or limbs, hyperplastic gonitis, etc.

2. Pinching-grasping

Manipulation: Apply strength to a selected area through the bellies of the thumb and middle fingers. Pinch and grasp the locale clockwise or anticlockwise (Fig. 83). It is recommended that there be pinching in grasping and vice versa, there be grasping in pinching. It be performed skillfully and successively with soft, gentle, but deepening and penetrating force for 3—5 minutes.

Functions: Relax muscles and Tendons, promote Blood circulation, relieve spasm and convulsion to stop pain, eliminate overfatigue.

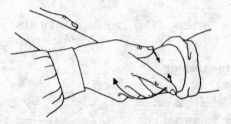

Fig. 83   Pinching-grasping

Indications: Soreness, pain, numbness, difficulty in flexing and extending of the neck, shoulder, and limbs.

3. Stroking-grasping (Benefiting the Brain)

Manipulation: Stand before the patient who is sitting. Support his (her) head with one hand, and stroke it with the five branched-off fingers of the other hand, from the anterior hairline to the posterior. The stroking actions should be performed on the left, the right and the middle part of the head in turn respectively, each for 10 times or so (Fig. 84). If patient's hair is long, wrap the hair up with a scarf or something like that before derigation. Having done this, rub Fengchi (GB 20) with the minor polythenar eminences by opening and shutting of the crossed hands for 5—10 times. Finally, grasp the skin of the head more than 10 times. This method is especially beneficial to the brain, thus also called Benefiting the Brain.

Functions: Tonify the brain, ease mental strain, refresh the mind, strengthen the Kidney, relieve Exterior Syndrome, expel Pathogenic Cold, restore Yang from collapse, induce resuscitation, relieve spasm and convulsion to stop pain.

Indications: Dizziness and vertigo, headache, migraine, common cold due to affection of exogenous Wind, Prostration Syndrome, syncope, loss of consciousness, lassitude, listlessness, neurosism, insomnia, amnesia, pain in the superciliary arch, tinnitus, deafness.

42

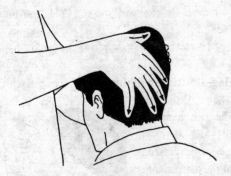

Fig. 84 Stoking-grasping (Benefiting the Brain)

4. Pushing-wiping

Manipulation: Support the head of the patient who is sitting on a chair with one hand, and apply strength through the lateral aspect of the thumb of the other hand. Perform pushing and wiping actions from the forehead to the area posterior to the patient's ear along the hairline at a high speed (Fig. 85). Operate on the left side first, then the right side, either for more than 10 times.

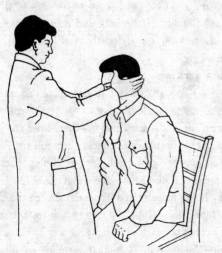

Fig. 85 Pushing-wiping

43

Functions: Subdue hyperactivity of the Liver and check its exuberant Yang, remove Pathogenic Wind and Cold, tranquilize and refresh the mind.

Indications: Headache, dizziness, common cold, hypertension, etc.

5. Opening-shutting-rubbing

Manipulation: Cross the fingers of the two hands to form an arc, and attach it closely to a diseased protruding portion of the patient. Manipulate by rubbing through the opening and shutting of the two palms until the patient perceives a local burning sensation resulted from the rapid and rhythmical rubbing force (Fig. 86).

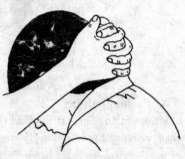

Fig. 86   Opening-shutting-rubbing

Functions: Warm and clear the Channels and Collaterals, dispel Pathogenic Wind and Cold, and promote the flow of Qi and Blood.

Indications: Rigidity of the neck and nape, headache caused by common cold, cervical spondylopathy, stiff-neck, traumatic knee joints, gonitis, etc.

6. Pulling-jerking

Manipulation: Ask the patient to lie supine and relax his (her) whole body completely. Hold the area above the ankle of the diseased side with the two hands, flex his (her) knee and hip joint forwards to his (her) chest several times, then pull the leg backwards and jerk it suddenly and powerfully for 1—2 times. Perform the manipulation on either limb in the same way (Fig. 87).

Functions: Relax muscles and Tendons, dredge the Channels and Collaterals, lubricate stiff joints, restore and treat injured soft tissues and dislocated bones.

Indications: Malposition in lumbar vertebrae, prolapse of intervertebral disc, etc.

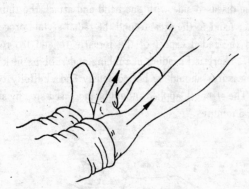

Fig. 87   Pulling-jerking

7. Kneading-pinching

Manipulation: Stand by the patient who is sitting. Hold his (her) elbow with one hand, knead and pinch his (her) shoulder along the biceps muscle and brachial triceps muscle up and down repeatedly (Fig. 88). The actions of kneading and pinching should be incorporated into an integrate action, and the strength increased gradually. Never be brutal. Repeat the actions for 3—5 minutes.

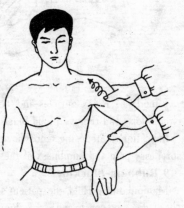

Fig. 88   Kneading-pinching

Functions: Relax muscles and Tendons, clear the Channels and Collaterals, activate Blood flow and alleviate pain.

Indications: Omalgia, arthralgia in the shoulder and arm, dysfunction of the shoulder joint.

8. Rubbing-kneading

Manipulation: Ask the patient to sit on a chair. Hold his (her) hand of the diseased side with one hand and attach the thumb belly of the other hand to the area around the radial styloid process. Rub and knead the radial aspect of the forearm to and fro repeatedly (Fig. 89). There is kneading in rubbing and rubbing in kneading; the two measures should be harmoniously and skillfully combined into one. The strength applied should be increased step by step. Repeat it 2—3 minutes.

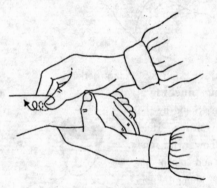

Fig. 89   Rubbing-kneading

Functions: Relax muscles and Tendons to smooth Qi and Blood circulation, and remove Blood Stasis and assuage pain.

Indications: Stenosing tenosynovitis in the radial styloid process, soreness, pain and numbness of the forearm.

9 Rubbing-plucking

Manipulation: Hold the patient's hand with one hand; rub his (her) diseased locale with the thumb or index finger of the other hand back and forth for several times; then pluck the lump with the thumb tip in various directions for 5—10 times (Fig. 90). The strength applied should be from mild to heavy, then from heavy to mild again.

Functions: Promote the subsidence of swelling, dissolve masses, detach adhesion, restore and treat the injured soft tissues.

Indications: Aponeurositis, sthcal cyst, painful lumps, subcutaneous nodules, etc.

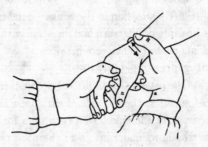

Fig. 90 Rubbing-plucking

10. Pulling the Legs while Pressing the Waist

Manipulation: Stand beside the patient, who lies prone with his (her) body relaxed and both hands holding the bedside. Ask an assistant to fix the patient's armpits and another assistant holds his (her) ankles, then stretch his (her) body by pulling in powerfully and persistently opposite directions. At this moment press his (her) lumbar region downwards strenuously with the overlapped palms for 10－20 times (Fig. 91). The strength applied should be gradually increased. It is contraindicated to release the patient's ankles suddenly and brutally after manipulation lest the patient's morbid condition become serious.

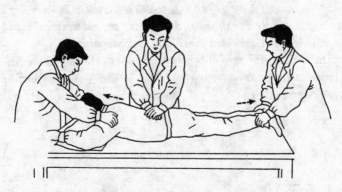

Fig. 91 Pulling the Legs while Pressing the Waist

47

Functions: Relax muscles and Tendons, clear and activate the Channels and Collaterals, correct deformity, help form intervertebral space and relieve oppression in the lumbar vertebrea.

Indications: Prolapse of intervertebral disc, synovial incarceration of the minor joints in the lumbar vertebrae, etc.

11. Kneading-pressing-vibrating

Manipulation: The patient lies on his (her) on a therapeutic bed. The practitioner stands at the left side. First, press and knead the patient's lower waist or the muscles on both sides for 5 — 6 times. Then, put several pillows under his (her) chest and pelvis to make the body higher. Press and vibrate the lumbar region with the overlapped palms for 10 — 20 times (Fig. 92). The strength applied should be gradually increased, and the manipulation scope enlarged step by step. It is contraindicated to give brutal actions.

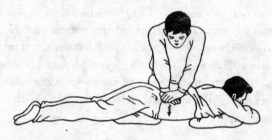

Fig. 92   Kneading-pressing-vibrating

Functions: Relieve muscular rigidity, restore and treat the injured soft tissues and dislocated joints in the lumbar vertebrae.

Indications: Prolapse of intervertebral disc, deformity of the posterior processes, hyperosteogeny of the lumbar vertebrae, lumbar muscle strain, etc.

POINTS
COMMONLY USED

*T*he so-called point refers to " Shu point", in which "Shu" means transferring in Chinese and "point" means an opening or a hole. Altogether three types of points have been classified. They are points on the Fourteen Regular Channels, extrachannel-points, and tender spots (Ashi points) (Fig. 93 – 95). The Fourteen Regular Channels are distributed on the traveling routes of the Twelve Regular Channels, Du Channel and Ren Channel. It is recorded that there are altogether 361 points in the human body. Extrachannel-points, which were later identified and nominated, occupy certain positions on the surface of the human body, yet do not belong to the traditional Fourteen Regular Channels. Tender spots, also called Ashi points, are non-fixed pressure pain points.

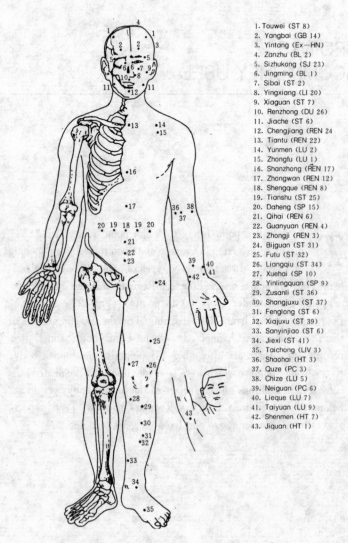

1. Touwei (ST 8)
2. Yangbai (GB 14)
3. Yintang (Ex—HN)
4. Zanzhu (BL 2)
5. Sizhukong (SJ 23)
6. Jingming (BL 1)
7. Sibai (ST 2)
8. Yingxiang (LI 20)
9. Xiaguan (ST 7)
10. Renzhong (DU 26)
11. Jiache (ST 6)
12. Chengjiang (REN 24
13. Tiantu (REN 22)
14. Yunmen (LU 2)
15. Zhongfu (LU 1)
16. Shanzhong (REN 17)
17. Zhongwan (REN 12)
18. Shengque (REN 8)
19. Tianshu (ST 25)
20. Daheng (SP 15)
21. Qihai (REN 6)
22. Guanyuan (REN 4)
23. Zhongji (REN 3)
24. Bijguan (ST 31)
25. Futu (ST 32)
26. Liangqiu (ST 34)
27. Xuehai (SP 10)
28. Yinlingquan (SP 9)
29. Zusanli (ST 36)
30. Shangjuxu (ST 37)
31. Fenglong (ST 6)
32. Xiajuxu (ST 39)
33. Sanyinjiao (ST 6)
34. Jiexi (ST 41)
35. Taichong (LIV 3)
36. Shaohai (HT 3)
37. Quze (PC 3)
38. Chize (LU 5)
39. Neiguan (PC 6)
40. Lieque (LU 7)
41. Taiyuan (LU 9)
42. Shenmen (HT 7)
43. Jiquan (HT 1)

Fig. 93   Points on the Front of the Human Body

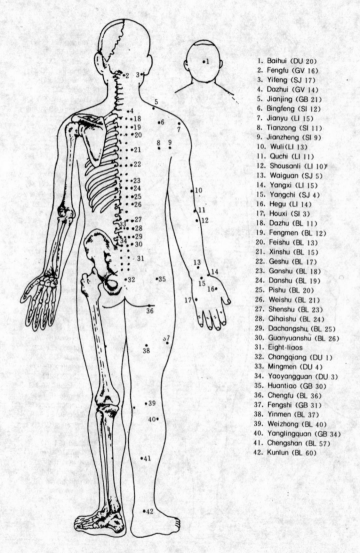

1. Baihui (DU 20)
2. Fengfu (GV 16)
3. Yifeng (SJ 17)
4. Dazhui (GV 14)
5. Jianjing (GB 21)
6. Bingfeng (SI 12)
7. Jianyu (LI 15)
8. Tianzong (SI 11)
9. Jianzheng (SI 9)
10. Wuli (LI 13)
11. Quchi (LI 11)
12. Shousanli (LI 10)
13. Waiguan (SJ 5)
14. Yangxi (LI 15)
15. Yangchi (SJ 4)
16. Hegu (LI 14)
17. Houxi (SI 3)
18. Dazhu (BL 11)
19. Fengmen (BL 12)
20. Feishu (BL 13)
21. Xinshu (BL 15)
22. Geshu (BL 17)
23. Ganshu (BL 18)
24. Danshu (BL 19)
25. Pishu (BL 20)
26. Weishu (BL 21)
27. Shenshu (BL 23)
28. Qihaishu (BL 24)
29. Dachangshu (BL 25)
30. Guanyuanshu (BL 26)
31. Eight-liaos
32. Changqiang (DU 1)
33. Mingmen (DU 4)
34. Yaoyangguan (DU 3)
35. Huantiao (GB 30)
36. Chengfu (BL 36)
37. Fengshi (GB 31)
38. Yinmen (BL 37)
39. Weizhong (BL 40)
40. Yanglingquan (GB 34)
41. Chengshan (BL 57)
42. Kunlun (BL 60)

Fig. 94   Points on the Back of the Human Body

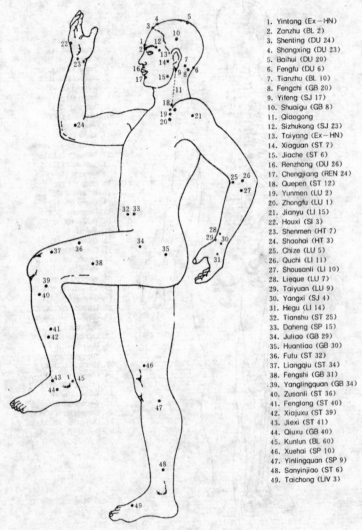

1. Yintang (Ex—HN)
2. Zanzhu (BL 2)
3. Shenting (DU 24)
4. Shangxing (DU 23)
5. Baihui (DU 20)
6. Fengfu (DU 6)
7. Tianzhu (BL 10)
8. Fengchi (GB 20)
9. Yifeng (SJ 17)
10. Shuaigu (GB 8)
11. Qiaogong
12. Sizhukong (SJ 23)
13. Taiyang (Ex—HN)
14. Xiaguan (ST 7)
15. Jiache (ST 6)
16. Renzhong (DU 26)
17. Chengjiang (REN 24)
18. Quepen (ST 12)
19. Yunmen (LU 2)
20. Zhongfu (LU 1)
21. Jianyu (LI 15)
22. Houxi (SI 3)
23. Shenmen (HT 7)
24. Shaohai (HT 3)
25. Chize (LU 5)
26. Quchi (LI 11)
27. Shousanli (LI 10)
28. Lieque (LU 7)
29. Taiyuan (LU 9)
30. Yangxi (SJ 4)
31. Hegu (LI 14)
32. Tianshu (ST 25)
33. Daheng (SP 15)
34. Juliao (GB 29)
35. Huantiao (GB 30)
36. Futu (ST 32)
37. Liangqiu (ST 34)
38. Fengshi (GB 31)
39. Yanglingquan (GB 34)
40. Zusanli (ST 36)
41. Fenglong (ST 40)
42. Xiajuxu (ST 39)
43. Jiexi (ST 41)
44. Qiuxu (GB 40)
45. Kunlun (BL 60)
46. Xuehai (SP 10)
47. Yinlingquan (SP 9)
48. Sanyinjiao (ST 6)
49. Taichong (LIV 3)

Fig. 95 Points on the Lateral of the Human Body

Measurement of
the Location of Points

The location methods often employed clinically are as follows: bone-length measurement (a method of locating acupoints by proportional length unit of the body), digital-proportion measurement, and natural-sign measurement.

Bone-length Measurement

1. Head

The length from the front hairline to the posterior hairline is defined as 12 cun; for those whose front hairline is not clear, the point is located 3 cun superior to the midpoint between the two eyebrows; for those whose posterior hairline not clear, the point is located 3 cun superior to Dazhui (DU 14); the length from the midpoint between the two eyebrows to Dazhui (DU 14) is defined as 18 cun. The length between the two papillary muscles on the back is defined as 9 cun.

2. Chest and Abdomen

The length between the two nipples is considered to be 8 cun; the length between the xiphosternal synchrodrosis to the navel is defined as 8 cun; the length between the navel and the upper margin of the public bone is defined as 5 cun.

3. Back

The length between the large pyramid and the caudal end is defined as 21 cun; the length between the spinal margin of the scapula to the middling of the back is defined as 3 cun.

4. Upper Limb

The length from the transverse crease of the anterior axilla to the transverse line of the elbow is defined as 9 cun; the length from the elbow transverse crease to that of the wrist is defined as 12 cun.

5. Lower Limb

At the medial aspect of the thigh, the length from the upper margin of the public bone to the condyle is defined as 18 cun; on the lateral side of the thigh, the length from the pertrochanteric to the popliteal fossa is defined as 19 cun.

At the medial aspect of the shank, the length from the tibia to the ankle is defined as 13 cun; at its the lateralaspect, the length from the lower margin of the knee-cap to the lateral ankle is defined as 16 cun.

Digital-proportion Measurement

1. Middle Finger
Flex the middle finger of the patient and the length of the middle segment of the flexed finger is defined as 1 cun.

2. Thumb
The width of the patient's thumb joint is taken as 1 cun.

3. Joined Fingers
Join all the fingers except the thumb together. The width of the four fingers, based on the middle digital transverse crease, is defined as 3 cun.

Natural Sign Measurement

Some natural signs on the human body, such as eyebrow, hairline, navel, nipple, nail, etc. can be considered as the signs to locate points in manipulation.

Head and Face

1. Jingming (BL 1)
Locale: 0.1 cun above the inner canthus (Fig. 96).

Manipulation: Support the patient's head with one hand, press or vibrate the point with the tip of a thumb or index finger of the other hand for 1—2 minutes.

Functions: Expel Pathogenic Wind and Heat, improve acuity of eyesight, and eliminate nebula.

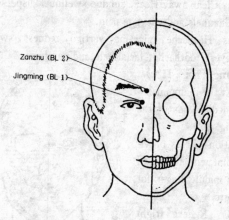

Fig. 96   Jingming (BL 1),Zanzhu (B2)

Indications: Myopia, blurred vision, redness, swelling and pain of eyes, irritated epiphora.

2. Zanzhu (BL 2)

Locale: At the medial end of the eyebrow (Fig. 96).

Manipulation: The same as the method mentioned-above

Functions: Tranquilize the mind, dispel Pathogenic Wind, clear away Heat, and improve acuity of sight.

Indications: Headache, pain in the superciliary arch, dizziness, blurred vision, flickering eyelid or blepharospasm. irritated epiphora.

3. Taiyang (Ex−HN)

Locale: In the depression 1 cun between the lateral end of the eyebrow and lateral canthi (Fig. 97).

Manipulation: Press and knead the point with the tips

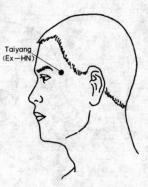

Fig. 97   Taiyand (Ex-HN)

of both middle fingers 30—50 times.

Functions: Clear away Heat, subdue swelling, disperse obstruction of the Channels and alleviate pain.

Indications: Headache, migraine, vertigo, redness, swelling and pain of the eyes, toothache, facial pain and paralysis.

4. Yintang (Ex—HN)

Locale: At the midpoint between the medial ends of the eyebrows(Fig. 98).

Manipulation: Press or vibrate the point with the tip of a thumb or middle finger for 0.5—1 minute.

Functions: Relieve fright and convulsion, ease mental stress, clear the eyes, and remove nasal obstruction.

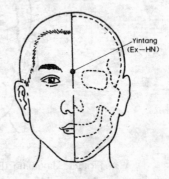

Fig. 98   Yintang (Ex-HN)

Indications: Insomnia, headache, vertigo, stuffy nose, and eye diseases.

5. Yingxiang (LI 20)

Locale: In the depression of the nasolabial groove, parallel to the lateral margin of the nose wing (Fig. 99).

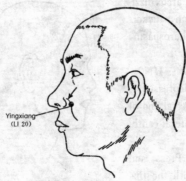

Fig. 99   Yingxiang (LI 20)

Manipulation: Press and knead either Yingxiang (LU 20) with the tips of the thumbs, or index fingers, or middle fingers of both hands for 30—50 times.

Functions: Disperse Wind, remove Heat, and eliminate nasal obstruction.

Indications: Stuffy watery nose, facial itching, rhinorrhea with turbid discharge, and facial paralysis.

6. Baihui (DU 20)

Locale: At the vertex of the head, a meeting point of the lines connecting both ear tips and the anterior and posterior hairlines(Fig. 100).

Manipulation: Support the patient's head with one hand, press and knead the point with the thumbnail of the other hand for 30—50 times.

Functions: Disperse Pathogenic Wind, refresh the mind, ascend Yang and arrest discharge.

Indications: Headache, vertigo, apoplexy, insomnia, amnesia, dysphasia, hemiplegia, prolapse of the rectum or uterus, and stuffy nose.

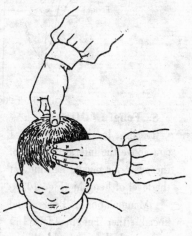

Fig. 100   Baihui (DU 20)

7. Fengchi (GB 20)

Locale: In the depression below the occipital bone, at the level of Fengfu (DU 16) (Fig. 101).

Manipulation: Press the point with the thumbtips or grasp the points with the bellies of the thumb and index finger of both hands.

Functions: Dispel Pathogenic Wind, remove endogenic Heat, and relieve Exterior Syndrome.

Indications: Headache, vertigo, stiff and painful neck, common cold, redness and pain of the eyes.

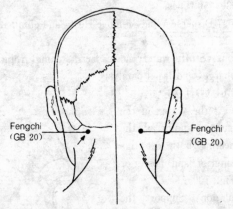

Fengchi
(GB 20)

Fengchi
(GB 20)

Fig. 101   Fengchi (GB 20)

8. Fengfu (DU 16)

Locale: In the depression 1 cun above the inferior margin of the posterior middle hairline, at the level of Fengchi (Fig. 102).

Manipulation: Press and knead either Fengfu (DU 16) with the bellies of both thumbs or middle fingers for 20 — 30 times.

Functions: Expel Pathogenic Wind.

Indications: Headache caused by Wind and Cold, stiffness and pain in the neck, cervical spondylopathy, dizziness, etc.

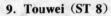

Fengfu
(DU 16)

Fig. 102   Fengfu (DU 16)

9. Touwei (ST 8)

Locale: At the angle between the two hairlines at the front (Fig. 103).

58

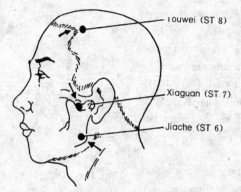

Fig. 103   Touwei (ST 8), Xiaguan (ST 7), Jiache (ST 6)

Manipulation: The same as mentioned-above.

Functions: Alleviate pain, improve acuity of sight, calm endopathic Wind, and arrest convulsion and spasm.

Indications: Headache, dizziness, ophthalmalgia, dizziness, blurred vision, irritated epiphora, blepharospasm.

10. Xiaguan (ST 7)

Locale: In the depression inferior to the zygomatic border and anterior to the mandibular condyloid process (Fig. 103).

Manipulation: The same as that of Fengfu mentioned-above.

Functions: Promote subsidence of swelling to assuage pain, clear the Channels and improve hearing.

Indications: Toothache, prosopodynia, deafness, tinnitus, disorder of mandibular joints, facial paralysis, and facial edema.

11. Jiache (ST 6)

Locale: At the protruding spot of the masseter when one clenches his teeth, close to the angle of the mandible (Fig. 103).

Manipulation: The same as that of Fengfu (DU 16) mentioned-above.

Functions: Disperse Wind, remove Heat, relieve stiff joints, and dredge the Channels.

Indications: Toothache, pain of the cheek, parotitis, trismus, rigidity and pain in the neck, facial paralysis.

12. Tinggong (SI 19)

Locale: Between the tragus and the mandibular joint, corresponding to the depression in front of the ear when one opens his mouth (Fig. 104).

Manipulation: Knead the point with the bellies of both middle fingers for 30 — 50 time.

Functions: Improve hearing and subdue swelling.

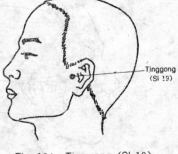

Fig. 104 Tinggong (SI 19)

Indications: Tinnitus, deafness, toothache and epilepsy.

13. Yuyao (Ex—HN)

Locale: At the midpoint of the eyebrow, directly above the pupil (Fig. 105).

Manipulation: Press and knead either point with the thumb bellies or tips of middle fingers of both hands 20 — 30 times.

Functions: Improve acuity of vision, subdue swelling, relieve rigidity of muscles and Tendons,

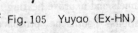

Fig. 105 Yuyao (Ex-HN)

and smooth the flow of Qi and Blood in the Channels and Collaterals.

Indications: Pain in the superciliary arch, redness, swelling and pain of the eyes, nebula, blepharoptosis and blepharospasm.

Back and Waist

1. Tianzong (SI 11)

60

Locale: In the infraspinous fossa, 0.5－1 cun inferior to the middle margin along the spinal scapula (Fig. 106).

Manipulation: Press the point with the radial interphalangeal joint of a thumb or its tip for 0.5－1 minute.

Functions: Relax muscles and Tendons, activate the flow of Qi and Blood in the Channels and Collaterals.

Indications: Pain in the scapular region and posterolateral part of the elbow and shoulder, fibrositis in back muscles, stiffneck, and cervical spondylopathy.

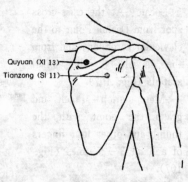

Fig. 106 Tianzong (SI 11), Quyuan (SI 13)

2. Quyuan (SI 13)

Locale: In the depression located on the medial and superior portion of the spine of the scapula (Fig. 106).

Manipulation: Press the point with the tip of a thumb or middle finger 0.5－1 minute.

Functions: The same as those of Tianzong (SI 11) mentioned-above.

Indications: Soreness and pain in the scapula, traumatic tissues in the back.

3. Dazhui (DU 14)

Locale: In the depression inferior to the spinous process of the 7th cervical vertebra (Fig. 107).

Manipulation: Press and knead the point with the belly of a thumb or middle finger.

Functions: Remove Heat from the body surface, prevent attack of malaria and epilepsy.

Indication: Stiffness, Cold and Heat of the neck, rigidity and pain of the back, nausea due to excessive Heat, vomiting, epilepsy, etc.

4. Jianjing (GB 21)

Locale: At the csiss-cross spot from Dazhui Point to the clavicular acromion, and from the clavicle to the spinal scapula (Fig. 107).

Manipulation: Pinch and grasp the point with the thumb and other four fingers of a hand 3 — 5 times (Fig. 107).

Functions: Expel Pathogenic Wind , remove Heat, subdue swelling and alleviate pain.

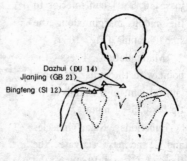

Fig. 107　Dazhui (DU 14), Jianjing (GB 21), Bingfeng (SI 12)

Indications: Arthralgia in the scapular and back regions, rigidity of the arms, stiffness and pain in the neck, general debility, apoplexy, and mastitis.

5. Bingfeng (SI 12)

Locale: At the center of the superior-scapular fossa, corresponding to the spot directly superior to Tianzong and 1 cun above the midpoint border of the spinal scapulae (Fig. 107).

Manipulation: Press and knead the point with the belly of a thumb or middle finger 20—30 times.

Functions: Relax muscles and Tendons, and expel Pathogenic Wind.

Indications: Rigidity and pain in the scapula, aching numbness of the upper limbs, traumatic tissues in the back, fibrositis, cervical spondylopathy, and stiffneck.

6. Jianzhongshu (SI 15)

Locale: 2 cun lateral to the spinal process of the 7th cervical vertebra (Fig. 108).

Manipulation: Press the point with the radial interphalangeal joint of a crooked thumb or the tip of the thumb for 0. 5—1 minute.

Functions: Relieve Exterior Syndrome, and ventilate the Lung.

Indications: Cough caused by common cold, fever, aversion to cold, pain in the back and neck, cervical spondylopathy.

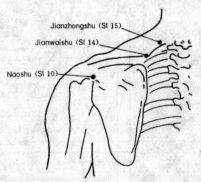

Fig. 108 Jianzhongshu (SI 15), Jianwaishu
(SI 14), Naoshu (SI 10)

7. Jianwaishu (SI 14)

Locale: 3 cun lateral to the spinal process of the 1st thoracic vertebra (Fig. 108).

Manipulation: The same as that of Jianzhongshu (SI 15) mentioned above.

Functions: Relax muscles and Tendons, smooth the flow of Qi and Blood in the Channels and Collaterals.

Indications: Soreness and pain in the shoulder and back, stiffness of the neck, cold and pain of the upper extremities.

8. Naoshu (SI 10)

Locale: In the depression inferioposterior to the prominence of the scapular acromion on the upper part of the shoulder (Fig. 108).

Manipulation: Press and knead the point with the belly of a thumb or middle finger for 0.5—1 minute.

Functions: Relax muscles and Tendons, promote the flow of Qi and Blood, arrest phlegm, and subdue swelling.

Indications: Soreness, pain and flaccidity of the shoulder and arm, omalgia, scrofula of the neck.

9. Fengmen (BL 12)

Locale: 1.5 cun lateral to the spinous process of the 2nd thoracic vertebra (Fig. 109).

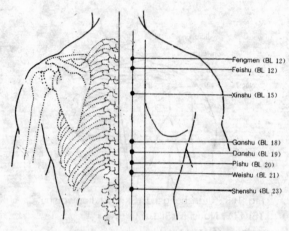

Fig. 109   Fengmen (BL 12), Feishu
(BL 13), Xinshu (BL 15) Ganshu
(BL 18),Danshu (BL 19), Pishu (BL 20),
Weishu (BL 21), Shenshu(BL 23)

Manipulation: Press either Fengmeng (BL 12) with the thumb tips for 0.5—1 minute.

Functions: Relieve Exterior Syndrome, facilitate the flow of Lung Qi, protect wei system, and strengthen the body surface resistance.

Indications: Nasal obstruction caused by common cold, cough due to Pathogenic Wind, headache, nasal discharge, chronic rhinitis, rigidity of the neck, and backache.

10. Feishu (BL 13)

Locale: 1.5 cun lateral to the lower border of the spinous process of the 3rd thoracic vertebra (Fig. 109).

Manipulation: Press and knead either Feishu (BL 13) with both thumb tips, or the pads of the index or middle fingers 30—50 times.

Functions: Relieve Exterior Syndrome to free the Lung and send down the ascending Lung Qi.

64

Indications: Cough due to common cold, stuffy nose, oppressed sensation in the chest, asthma, pneumonia, aching pain in the back, hectic fever due to Yin Deficiency, night sweat.

11. Xinshu (BL 15)

Locale: 1.5 cun lateral to the lower border of the spinous process of the 5th thoracic vertebra (Fig. 109).

Manipulation: Press and knead either point with the pads of both thumbs, or index and middle fingers 50—100 times.

Functions: Tranquilize the mind and relieve mental stress, soothe the chest oppression, and send down the upward adverse flow of Qi.

Indications: Insomnia, amnesia, palpitation, vexation, nocturnal emission, stenocardia, chest pain radiating to the back, heart diseases such as arrhythmia, etc.

12. Ganshu (BL 18)

Locale: 1.5 cun lateral to the lower border of the spinous process of the 9th thoracic vertebra (Fig. 109).

Manipulation: The same way as that of Xinshu mentioned-above.

Functions: Soothe the Liver, normalize the functions of the Gallbladder, relieve mental stress, and promote acuity of sight.

Indications: Pain in chest and hypochondrium, insomnia, lumbago, backache, myopia, optic atrophy, hepatopathy, cholecystopathy, and gastropathy.

13. Danshu (BL 19)

Locale: 1.5 cun lateral to the lower border of the spinous process of the 10th thoracic vertebra (Fig. 109).

Manipulation: Press the point with both thumbs 1—2 minutes.

Functions: Dispel Heat and remove Dampness, normalize secretion of the Gallbladder, and alleviate pain.

Indications: Distress and pain in the hypochondriac region, bitter taste, dry mouth, hepatopathy, cholecystopathy, and spasm of esophagus.

14. Pishu (BL 20)

Locale: 1.5 cun lateral to the lower border of the spinous process of the 11th thoracic vertebra (Fig. 109).

Manipulation: The same way as that of Danshu (BL 19).

Functions: Invigorate the Spleen, relieve Dampness, send up essential substances, and arrest diarrhea.

Indications: abdominal distention, protracted diarrhea, hypochondriac pain, jaundice, edema, indigestion, insomnia, pneumonia, malaria, swelling and pain of the Spleen, amen, edema, chronic Wind Syndrome of the Spleen.

15. Weishu (BL 21)

Locale: 1.5 cun lateral to the lower border of the spinous process of the 12th thoracic vertebra or the upper border of the 1st lumbar vertebra (Fig. 109).

Manipulation: The same way as that of Danshu.

Functions: Normalize the functions of the Stomach, Spleen and the Middle Jiao, and send down adverse rising of Qi.

Indications: epigastralgia, abdominal distention, vomiting, protracted diarrhea, indigestion.

16. Shenshu (BL 23)

Locale: 1.5 cun lateral to the lower border of the spinous process of the 2nd lumbar vertebra (Fig. 109).

Manipulation: The same way as that of Danshu (BL 19).

Functions: Tonify Kidney Yang, improve inspiration, and induce diuresis.

Indications: lumbago due to Kidney Deficiency, soreness and pain of the loins and knees, seminal emission, enuresis, impotence, thamuria, irregular menstruation, tinnitus, and deafness.

17. Mingmen (DU 4)

Locale: At the depression inferior to the spinous process of the 2nd lumbar vertebra (Fig. 110).

Manipulation: Rub the point with the entire palm of a hand until a local warm sensation is perceived by the patient.

Functions: Warm and recuperate Kidney Yang, relax muscles and Tendons, relieve convulsion and spasm.

Indications: Soreness, pain and weakness of the waist, seminal emission, tinnitus, thamuria, abdominal pain, headache, fever, leukorrhea with reddish discharge, arthralgia due to Cold.

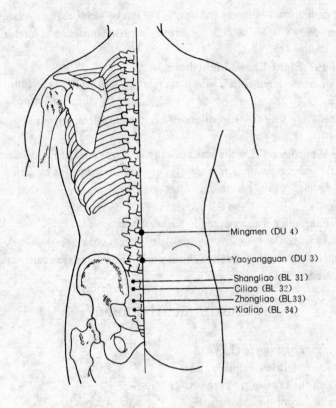

Fig. 110   Mingmen (DU 4), Yaoyangguan (DU 3),
Eight-liaos: Shangliao (BL 31), Ciliao (BL 32),
Zhongliao (BL 33), Xialiao (BL 34)

18. Yaoyangguan (DU 3)

Locale: In the depression inferior to the spinous process of the
4th lumbar vertebra (Fig. 110).

Manipulation: Press and knead the point with the pad of a thumb
or a palm for 0.5—1 minute. Good results will be obtained when
the patient perceives a warm sensation on the locale.

Functions: Remove Cold and Dampness, relax muscles and Tendons, and free the flow of Qi and Blood in the Channels and Collaterals.

Indications: Soreness and pain in the lumbo-sacral region, sprain and muscle strain in the waist, hyperplastic inflammation of lumbar vertebrae.

19. Eight-liaos (Eight-holes)

Locale: Eight-liaos , which contain Shangliao (BL 31), Ciliao (BL 32), Zhongliao (BL 33), and Xialiao (BL 34), locate in the 1st, 2nd, 3rd, and 4th posterior sacral foramens respectively (Fig. 110).

Manipulation: Let the patient lie prone. Press and dot Eight-liaos (B31-34) 5-6 times respectively, or manipulate by rubbing with a palm until a local penetrating warm sensation is perceived by the patient.

Functions: Warm and tonify Kidney Yang.

Indications: lumbago, soreness and pain in the sacral region, seminal emission, impotence, difficulty in urination, dysmenorrhea, amenorrhea.

Chest and Abdomen

1. Zhangmen (LIV 13)

Locale: Below the lower border of the floating rib at the lateral aspect of the abdomen (Fig. 111).

Manipulation: Press and knead both points with the pads of both thumbs or middle fingers 30-50 times.

Functions: Strengthen the Spleen, relieve flatulence, normalize the functions of the Stomach and Gallbladder.

Indications: Abdominal pain and distention, borborygmus,

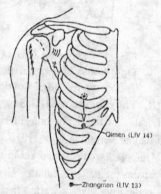

Qimen (LIV 14)

Zhangmen (LIV 13)

Fig. 111 Zhangmen (LIV 13), Qimen (LIV 14)

diarrhea, vomiting, pain in the chest and hypochondrium, listlessness, lassitude of limbs, jaundice, Cold and pain along the spinal column, masses in the abdomen.

2. Qimen (LIV 14)

Locale: At the 6th intercostal space straightly below the nipple (Fig. 111).

Manipulation: The same as mentioned-above in Zhangmen (LIV 13).

Functions: Soothe the Liver, strengthen the Spleen, regulate the Stomach, and check the upward adverse flow of Qi.

Indications: Fullness and pain in the chest and hypochondrium, vomiting, hiccup, acid regurgitation, abdominal distention, diarrhea, cough with dyspnea.

3. Guanyuan (REN 4)

Locale: 3 cun below the umbilicus along the middle line of the abdomen (Fig. 112).

Manipulation: Let the patient lie supine. Press it with the pad of a thumb or middle finger, then knead it along the breathing wave of the patient for 1—2 minutes. The strength applied should be soft, gentle, deepening and penetrating.

Functions: Reinforce and invigorate Vital Qi, treat scanty and dark urine, and also stranguria.

Indications: Seminal emission, impotence, irregular menstruation, amenorrhea, dysmenorrhea, prolapse of the uterus or rectum, leukorrhea with reddish discharge, metrorrhagia and metrostaxis, vertigo, thamuria, anuresis, and nebulous urine.

4. Qihai (REN 6)

Locale: 1.5 cun below the umbilicus (Fig. 112).

Manipulation: The same way as mentioned-above.

Functions: Strengthen Qi and Yang, regulate menstruation, and arrest spontaneous emission.

Indications: Irregular menstruation, amenorrhea dysmenorrhea, prolapsed uterus or rectum, leukorrhea with reddish discharge, metrorrhagia and metrostaxis, dysmenorrhea, amenorrhea, leukorrhea, dizziness, diarrhea, impotence, lassitude of limbs, emaciation, and indigestion.

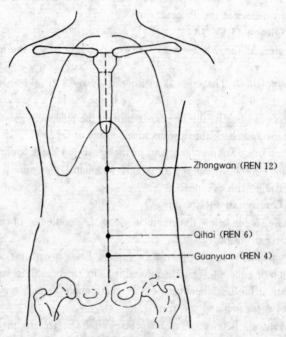

Zhongwan (REN 12)

Qihai (REN 6)

Guanyuan (REN 4)

Fig. 112 Guanyuan (REN 4), Qihai (REN 6),
Zhongwan (REN 12)

5. Zhongwan (REN 12)

Locale: 4 cun below the umbilicus, correspondingly at the mid-point between the lower end of the sternum and the umbilicus (Fig. 112).

Manipulation: Let the patient lie supine with his (her) lower limbs flexed naturally. Rub the point with a palm for 3—5 minutes; or press the point with the middle finger for 1—2 minutes.

Functions: Regulate the Stomach, strengthen the Spleen, promote the flow of Qi and send down its upward adverse flow.

Indications: Epigastalgia, abdominal distention, loss of appetite, vomiting, hiccup, acid regurgitation, borborygmus, diarrhea, insomnia, asthma, palpitation due to fright.

70

Upper Limbs

1. Hegu (LI 4)

Locale: Between the 1st and 2nd metacarpal bones on the dorsum of the hand, close to the midpoint of the second metacarpal bone of the radial side (Fig. 113).

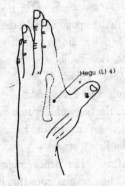

Fig. 113   Hegu (LI 4)

Manipulation: Press and knead the point with the tip of a thumb 20—30 times.

Functions: Clear away Pathogenic Heat from the body surface, and promote acuity of sight and hearing.

Indications: Headache, vertigo, redness, swelling and pain of eyes, rhinorrhea with turbid discharge, epistaxis, toothache, deafness, facial edema, sore-throat, stiff mandible, facial paralysis, mumps, spasm and pain of the upper extremities, hemiplegia, chills, fever, stomachache, abdominal pain, amenorrhea, and constipation.

2. Yangxi (LI 5)

Locale: In the fossa between the tendon of M. extensor pollicis longus and tendon of m. extensor pollicis brevis on the radial side of the wrist (Fig. 114).

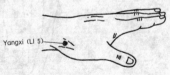

Fig. 114   Yangxi (LI 5)

Manipulation: The same as mentioned-above.

Functions: Remove Pathogenic Heat, refresh the mind, improve eyesight, and relieve sorethroat.

71

Indications: Headache, deafness, tinnitus, sore-throat, toothache, eye diseases such as conjunctival congestion, pain in the upper limbs.

3. Lieque (LU 7)

Locale: 1. 5 cun above the wrist transverse crease of the radial side, correspondingly at the spot the index finger reaches when the two hands are criss-crossed (Fig. 115).

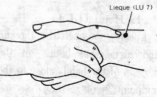

Fig. 115   Lieque (LU 7)

Manipulation: Press and knead it with the belly of a thumb or its lateral tip 20—30 times.

Functions: Ventilate the Lung, dispel exopathy, remove obstruction in the Ren Channel.

Indications: Headache, migraine, rigidity of the neck, facial paralysis, hemiplegia, sore-throat, cough, and dyspnea.

4. Shousanli (LI 10)

Locale: 2 cun below Quchi (LI 11) with the arm flexed, and on the connecting line between Yangxi and Quchi at the medial aspect of the radium (Fig. 116).

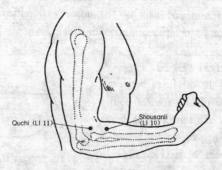

Fig. 116   Shousanli (LI 10), Quchi (LI 11)

Manipulation: Press and knead it with the belly of a thumb 30—50 times.

Functions: Remove Heat, promote acuity of vision, clear the

72

Channels and Collaterals to free the flow of Qi and Blood.

Indications: Abdominal distention, vomiting, diarrhea, toothache, swelling of cheeks, sudden loss of voice, hemiplegia, numbness, pain, and rigidity of the upper limbs, eye disorders.

5. Quchi (LI 11)

Locale: In the depression at the radial aspect of the elbow transverse crease when the elbow is flexed (Fig. 116).

Manipulation: The same way as it is done in Shousanli (LI 10).

Functions: Dispel Wind to arrest itching, remove Heat and swelling.

Indications: Swelling, pain, paralysis and weakness of the upper limbs, toothache, sore-throat, redness and pain of the eyes, distress and fullness in the chest, abdominal pain, diarrhea, irregular menstruation, etc.

6. Xiaohai (SI 8)

Locale: Between the triangular plane of the flexed elbow and the medial epicondyle of the humerus (Fig. 117).

Manipulation: Pluck the point softly with an index finger 3—5 times.

Functions: Relieve rigidity of muscles and Tendons, regulate Blood circulation, soothe the Liver, remove Heat, and ease mental stress.

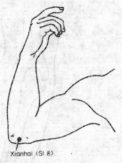

Xianhai (SI 8)

Fig. 117 Xiaohai (SI 8)

Indications: Pain of the neck or lateral side of the shoulder, swelling of the cheeks, headache, dizziness, impairment of hearing, tinnitus, soreness and swelling, and epilepsy.

7. Shaohai (HT 3)

Locale: In the depression at the ulnar aspect of the elbow transverse crease when the elbow is flexed (Fig. 118).

Manipulation: Press and knead it with the belly of a thumb or middle finger for 30—50 times.

73

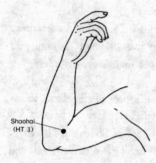

Functions: Relieve mental strain, and relax muscles and Tendons to free the flow of Qi and Blood in the Channels and Collaterals.

Indications: Precordial pain, insomnia, headache, dizziness, pain in the armpit and hypochondrium, numbness and tremor of the upper limbs, sudden loss of voice, mania, delirium, and scofula.

Fig. 118   Shaohai (HT 3)

8. Yangchi (SJ 4)

Locale: At the wrist transverse crease directly above the ring finger, corresponding to the depression on the back of the wrist (see Fig. 119).

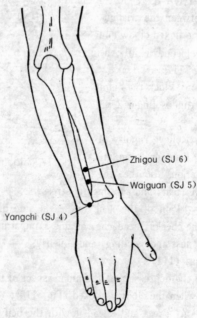

Fig. 119   Yangchi (SJ 4),
Waiguan (SJ 5), Zhigou (SJ 6)

Manipulation: The same as that of Shaohai (HT 3) mentioned-above.

Functions: Relax muscles and Tendons and activate the flow of Qi and Blood in the Channels and Collaterals, arrest sore-throat, improve hearing, treat diseases of both Exterior and Interior Syndrome. sprain in the wrist, pain of the shoulder and back, deafness, malaria, dire thirst, dry mouth, and sore-throat.

9. Waiguan (SJ 5)

Locale: In the depression between the radius and ulna, 2 cun above Yangchi Point (Fig. 119).

Manipulation: The same way as shown in Shaohai (HT 3).

Functions: Relieve Exterior Syndrome, and improve hearing and eyesight.

Indications: Affection by Cold, exogenous febrile diseases, headache, pain in the cheek, shoulder and back regions or fingers, rigidity of the arm and elbow, tremour of the hand, tinnitus, deafness, redness, swelling and pain of the eyes.

10. Zhigou (SJ 6)

Locale: In the depression between the radius and ulna, 3 cun above Yangchi Point (Fig. 119).

Manipulation: The same way as shown in Shaohai (HT 3).

Functions: Disperse Heat, improve hearing, lower the upward adverse flow of Qi, and loose the bowel.

Indications: Tinnitus, deafness, constipation, vomiting, hypochondriac pain, aching pain of the back and shoulder, sudden loss of voice, febrile diseases, etc.

11. Quze (PC 3)

Locale: In the depression of the elbow transverse line, corresponding to the ulnar end of the brachial biceps (Fig. 120).

Manipulation: Press and knead it with the belly of a thumb 20 — 30 times.

Functions: Disperse obstruction in the Channels, alleviate pain, refresh the mind, regulate the functions of the Stomach and check its regurgitation.

Indications: Pain of the upper limbs, precordial pain, gastralgia, palpitation, fright, vomiting, hemoptysis, febrile diseases, and fid-

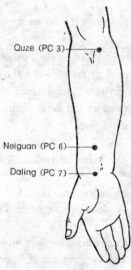

Quze (PC 3)

Neiguan (PC 6)

Daling (PC 7)

Fig. 120 Quze (PC 3),
Neiguan (PC 6), Daling
(PC7)

gets.

12. Neiguan (PC 6)

Locale: 2 cun above the mid-point of the wrist transverse crease at the medial aspect of the forearm (Fig. 120).

Manipulation: Press and knead it with the belly of a thumb or middle finger 30—50 times.

Functions: Relieve mental anxiety, assuage pain, soothe the Liver, and normalize the functions of the Stomach and Spleen.

Indications: Gapigastria, precordial pain, palpitation, insomnia, vomiting, contracture and pain of the upper limbs, epilepsy, febrile diseases, etc.

13. Daling (PC 7)

Locale: At the midpoint of the wrist transverse crease at the medial aspect of the forearm (Fig. 120).

Manipulation: As shown in Neiguan (PC 6).

Functions: Relieve mental stress, relax muscles and Tendons to alleviate pain, remove oppressed sensation in the chest, and normalize the functions of the Stomach and Spleen.

Indications: Precordial pain, wrist pain, mania, epilepsy, depressed emotions, cough with dyspnea, etc.

14. Binao (LI 14)

Locale: 7 cun above Quchi (LI 11), corresponding to the inferior end of the deltoid muscle at the radial aspect of the humerus (Fig. 121).

Manipulation: Press and knead Binao with the pad of a thumb for 20—30 times.

Functions: Regulate the flow of Qi, resolve phlegm, clear away

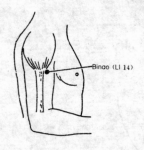

Fig. 121 Binao (LI 14)

Heat, and improve eyesight.

Indications: Pain in the shoulder and arm, rigidity of the neck, eye diseases, and scrofula.

15. Jianyu (LI 15)

Locale: At the corner of the shoulder (Fig. 122).

Manipulation: Press and knead Jianyu with the thumb tip or its flexed interphalangeal joint at the radial aspect for 0.5—1 minute.

Functions: Remove Pathogenic Wind and Heat, and resolve phlegm and itching.

Indications: Contracture and pain in the upper limbs, hemiplegia, eruption due to Pathogenic Wind and Heat, scrofula, and goiter in the neck.

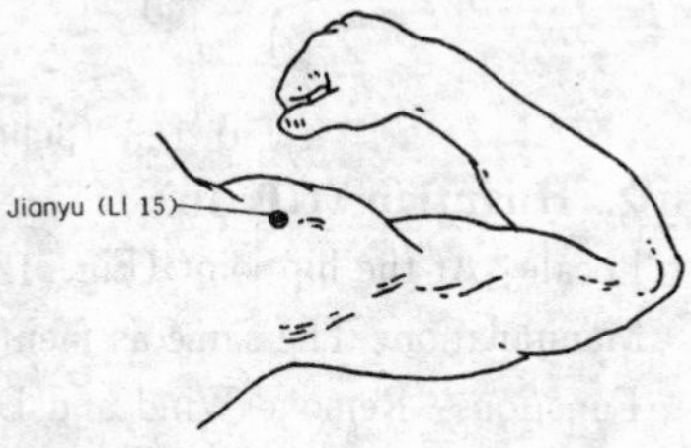

Fig. 122 Jianyu (LI 15)

Lower Limbs

1. Juliao (ST 3)

Locale: At the midpoint between the line of the anterosuperior iliacspine and the pertrochanteric prominence of the thigh (Fig. 123).

Manipulation: Ask the patient to lie on his (her) side. Press and knead the point with the thumb or the triangular plane of the flexed elbow for 0.5—1 minute.

Functions: Remove Pathogenic Wind and Dampness, relieve rigidity of muscles and joints, strengthen the waist and tonify the Kidney.

Indications: Pain in the lumbar region and hip, paralysis of the lower extremities, hernia.

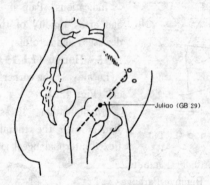

Fig. 123   Juliao (GB 29)

2. Huantiao (GB 30)

Locale: At the hip joint (Fig. 124).

Manipulation: The same as mentioned-above.

Functions: Remove Wind and Dampness, clear and activate the Channels and Collaterals.

Indications: Pain in the waist and hip, paralysis of the lower limbs, lumbago due to sudden sprain, swelling, pain and difficulty in turning the knee and ankle, hemiplegia, and general eruption.

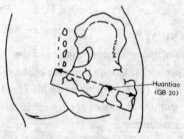

Fig. 124   Huantiao (GB 30)

3. Chengfu (BL 50)

Locale: At the midpoint of the gluteal transverse crease (Fig. 125).

Manipulation: Let the patient lie on his (her) back. Press and

78

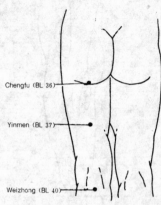

Chengfu (BL 36)

Yinmen (BL 37)

Weizhong (BL 40)

Fig. 125 Chengfu (BL 36),
Yinmen (BL 37), Weizhong
(BL 40)

knead (or dot) the point with the thumb tip or the triangular plane of the flexed elbow for 1 — 2 minutes.

Functions: Relax muscles and Tendons, activate the flow of Qi and Blood in the Channels and Collaterals, and treat hemorrhoids and constipation.

Indications: Pain in the lumbar, sacral, gluteal or femoral regions, hemorrhoids, and constipation.

4. Yinmen (BL 37)

Locale: About 6 cun below Chengfu, and on the line between Chengfu and Weizhong (Fig. 125).

Manipulation: The same as that of Chengfu (BL 50) mentioned-above.

Functions: Relax muscles and Tendons, smooth the flow of Qi and Blood in the Channels and Collaterals to ease pain.

Indications: Stiffness and pain along the spinal column, difficulty lying supine, pain of the thigh, etc.

5. Weizhung (BL 40)

Locale: At the midpoint of the transverse crease of the popliteal fossa (see Fig 125).

Manipulation: Let the patient flex his (her) knee naturally. Press the point with the thumb for 10—20 times, or grasp it 3—5 times.

Functions: Treat Blood disorders, promote subsidence of swelling, clear away Pathogenic Heat and clear the brain.

Indications: Lumbago, backache, disturbance of activities in the hip joint, contracture of popliteal tendons, paralysis in the lower limbs, abdominal pain, vomiting, dysuria, enuresis, apoplectic coma, nose-bleeding, furuncle, erysipelas, etc.

6. Fengshi (GB 31)

Locale: 7 cun above the popliteal transverse crease at the lateral aspect of the thigh, just the spot the middle finger tip reaches when one stands and droops his (her) arm (Fig. 126).

Manipulation: Press and knead the point with the thumb belly for 0. 5—1 minute.

Functions: Remove Pathogenic Wind and Dampness, dredge the Channels and Collaterals .

Indications: Hemiplegia due to apoplexy, paralysis of the lower extremities, general pruritus, and beriberi.

7. Yanglingquan (GB 34)

Locale: In the depression below the head of the fibula at the lateral aspect of the knee (Fig. 126).

Manipulation: The same as mentioned in Fengshi (GB 31).

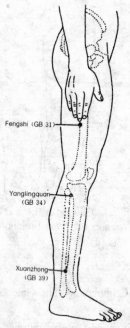

Fig. 126　Fengshi (GB 31), Yanglingquan (GB 34), Xuanzhong (GB 39)

Functions: Relax muscles and Tendons, relieve convulsion and spasm, soothe the Liver, and normalize the functions of the Gallbladder.

Indications: Paralysis of the lower limbs, swelling and pain of the knees, hemiplegia, hypochondriac pain, bitter taste, vomiting, and beriberi.

8. Xuanzhong (GB 39)

Locale: Above the lateral malleolus (Fig. 126).

Manipulation: The same as mentioned in Fengshi (GB 31).

Functions: Calm and soothe the Liver to stop endogeneous Wind, and tonify the Kidney.

Indications: Hemiplegia, stiffness and pain of the neck, distention and fullness in the chest and abdomen, hypochondriac pain, swelling at the armpit, pain of the lower limbs, apoplexy, and beriberi.

9. Biguan (ST 31)

Locale: At the femoral junction, opposite to Chengfu (Fig. 127).

Manipulation: The same as mentioned in Fengshi (GB 31).

Functions: Remove obstruction in the Channels and collatterals.

Indications: Flaccidity and arthralgia of the thigh, pain in the loins and lower limbs, and muscle contracture and numbness.

10. Futu (ST 32)

Locale: 6 cun above the laterosuperior margin of the patella, corresponding to the lateral muscle prominence above the patella (Fig. 127).

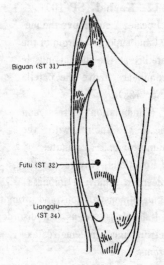

Fig. 127 Biguan (ST 31), Futu (ST 32), Liangqiu (ST 34)

Manipulation: The same as mentioned in Fengshi (GB 31).

Functions: Remove Pathogenic Cold and Dampness, dredge the Channels and Collaterals.

Indications: Pain in the waist and hip region, paralysis and Cold sensation in the lower limbs, beriberi, hernia, and abdominal distention.

11. Liangqiu (ST 34)

Locale: In the depression 2 cun above the lateralsuperior margin of the patella (Fig. 127).

Manipulation: The same as mentioned in Fengshi (GB 31).

Functions: Regulate the functions of the Stomach, arrest swelling, and tranquilize the mind to arrest pain.

Indications: Gastralgia, swelling and pain in the knee joint, and acute mastitis.

12. Xuehai (SP 10)

Locale: 2 cun above the medial and superior margin of the patella, at the medial muscle prominence above the patella (Fig. 128).

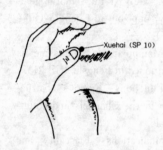

Fig. 128   Xuehai (SP 10)

Manipulation: Press and knead the point with the thumb for 0.5—1 minute.

Functions: Invigorate the Spleen to remove Dampness, regulate menstruation, and promote Blood circulation.

Indications: Menstrual disorders, dysmenorrhea, amenorrhea, metrorrhagia and metrostaxis, pain of the medial thigh, and eczema.

13 Dubi (Waixiyan) (ST 35)

Locale: At the external foramen below the kneecap (Fig. 129).

Manipulation: Press the point with the thumb at the radial aspect for 0.5—1 minute.

Functions: Remove Cold and Dampness, clear and activate the Channels and Collaterals, and relieve joint rigidity.

Indications: Swelling , pain and rigidity of the knee and patella, flaccidity of the lower extremeties, and beriberi.

14. Zusanli (ST 36)

Locale: 3 cun below the knee or Dubi Point (Fig. 129).

Manipulation Press and knead the point with the thumb for 1—2 minutes.

Functions: Strengthen the Spleen and Stomach, promote diges-

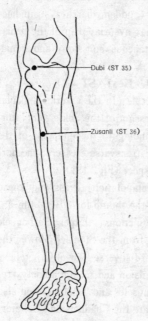

Fig. 129 Dubi (ST 35), Zusanli (ST 36)

tion, regulate Qi and Blood circulation, dispel Wind and remove Dampness, clear and activate the Channels and Collaterals, strengthen Defensive Qi and reinforce Vital Qi.

Indications: Gastralgia, nausea, vomiting, anorexia, abdominal distention and pain, borborygmi, diarrhea, indigestion, constipation, headache, dizziness, insomnia, tinnitus, consumptive diseases, apoplexy, cough, edema, dyspnea, beriberi, paralysis of the lower limbs, soreness and convulsion of the knee and tibia, and hemiplegia.

15. Sanyinjiao (SP 6)

Locale: 3 cun above the prominence of the medial malleolus (Fig. 130).

Manipulation: The same as mentioned-above.

Functions: Strengthen the Spleen, remove Dampness, regulate the functions of the Liver and Kidney.

Indications: Debility of the Spleen and Stomach, borborygmi, diarrhea, indigestion, irregular menstruation, metrorrhagia and metrostaxis, amenorrhea, prolapsed uterus, leukorrhea with reddish discharge, impotence, emission, dysuria, insomnia, testicular atrophy, edema, paralysis of the lower limbs, and eczema.

16 Yinlingquan (SP 9)

Locale: In the depression at the inferior margin of the medial epicondyle of the tibia (Fig. 130).

Manipulation: The same as mentioned in Zusanli.

Functions: Strengthen the Spleen, remove Dampness, Tonify the Kidney, and treat nocturnal emission.

83

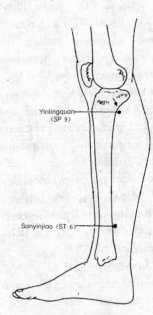

Yinlingquan
(SP 9)

Sanyinjiao (ST 6)

Fig. 130 Yinlingquan
(SP 9), Sanyinjiao
(ST 6)

Indications: Abdominal distention, sudden diarrhea, jaundice,
edema, dysuria, pain of the penis,
spontaneous emission, and gonal-
gia.

17. Jiexi (ST 41)

Locale: In the anterior articular
depression of the ankle joint, corresponding to the midpoint of the
ankle transverse crease at the dorsal aspect (Fig. 131).

Manipulation: Press and knead
with the thumb for 30—50 times.

Functions: Expel Pathogenic
Heat from the Stomach, lower the
upward adverse flow of Qi , relieve
convulsion and mental anxiety, relax muscles and Tendons, and also
activate the Channels and Collaterals.

Indications: Abdominal distention, constipation, delirium due to
Heat Syndrome of the Stomach, mania, conjunctival congestion,
headache, dizziness, pain in the superciliary arch, and sprain of the
ankle.

18. Chengshan (BL 57)

Locale: Below the two bellies of the gastrocnemius muscle (Fig.
132).

Manipulation: Press and knead the point with the thumb for 0. 5
—1 minute, or pinch and grasp it for 3—5 times.

Functions: Relax muscles and Tendons, regulate the flow of Qi to
alleviate pain, and treat hemorrhoids.

Indications: Systremma, lumbago, backache, abdominal pain,
constipation, epistaxis, hernia, hemorrhoids, and beriberi.

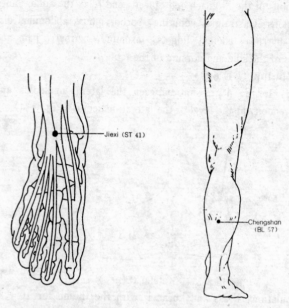

Fig. 131　Jiexi (ST 41)　Fig. 132　Chengshan (BL 57)

19. Gongsun (SP 4)

Locale: In the depression at the anterioinferior margin of the first metatarsal base, at the white skin of the big toe (Fig. 133).

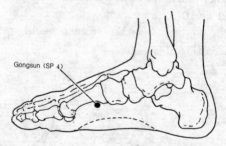

Fig. 133　Gongsun (SP 4)

Manipulation: Press and knead the point with the thumb for 0.5 — 1 minute.

Functions: Strengthen the Spleen, remove Dampness, normalize

85

the functions of the Stomach and Spleen, and relax the ankle joint.

Indications: Gastralgia, vomiting, borborygmus, abdominal distension, diarrhea, edema, fidgets, insomnia, beriberi, pain and numbness of the sole and dorsum of the foot.

20. Kunlun (BL 60)

Locale: In the depression between the lateral malleolus and Achilles tendon, at the level of the lateral malleolus (Fig. 134).

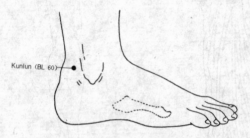

Kunlun (BL 60)

Fig. 134   Kunlun (BL 60)

Manipulation: Press and knead it with the thumb for 10 − 20 times.

Functions: Relieve convulsion to alleviate pain, arrest epilepsy, and remove Heat to prevent the attack of malaria.

Indications: Soreness and pain of the ankle joint, lumbago, backache, headache, pain in the neck, dystocia, and malaria.

21. Taixi (KID 3)

Locale: In the depression between the medial malleolus and Achilles tendon (Fig. 135).

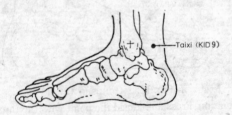

Taixi (KID 9)

Fig. 135   Taixi (KID 9)

Manipulation: The same as mentioned-above.

86

Functions: Invigorate Kidney Qi, and strengthen the Lung and Spleen.

Indications: Headache, dizziness, tinnitus, deafness, sorethroat, toothache, cough with dyspnea, irregular menstruation, insomnia, anemia, spermatorrhea, impotence, pain along the spinal column, frequent micturition, cold sensation in the lower limbs, swelling and pain of the medial malleolus.

COMMON DISEASES IN TUINA PRACTICE

Traumatology

Injury of Upper Limbs

1. External Humeral Epicondylitis

*E*xternal Humeral Epicondylitis, also known as tennis elbow, results mainly from frequent trauma and prolonged chronic strain at the extensor muscle point of the forearm.

Etiology and Pathogenesis

When the attaching point of extensor muscles of the laterosuperior humeral condyle, the ring ligaments, and the articular synovium of the humerus are damaged by external forces, there will occur the following pathological changes: ligamental fracture, circumscribed hyperemia, swelling and exudation of aseptic inflammation; consequently such changes as proliferation of fibrous tissues, organization, adhesion, etc.

Clinical manifestations

The onset begins with soreness and pain at the posterolateral elbow, radiating downwards along the extensor muscle of the fore-arm, slight local swelling, obvious tenderness and difficulty in turning the forearm or grasping with the hand. The pain is aggravated when the patient performs such actions as lifting, drawing, and pushing. The tennis elbow test shows positive, but the X-ray examination reveals no abnormal phenomena.

Tuina manoeuvres

Principal methods: Treat the disease by Rolling, Kneading with the Palm Base, Grasping, Plucking and Rubbing with Both Thenar Eminences.

Subordinate methods: Knead the tender spots, Quchi (LI 11), Shousanli (LI 10), Hegu (LI 4), and Quze (PC 3).

The treatment should be given once a day or every other day.

Case

Liu, female, 43, fitter. First visit: Dec. 6, 1988.

Symptoms: Pain in the right elbow for a month.

Case history: The patient was affected with soreness and pain at the right posterolateral elbow for a month because of overfatigue for work. The pain radiates downwards along the radial aspect of the forearm, and was aggravated even when she did light work like lifting a tea pot, twisting a towel, etc. As no oral administration of both Chinese and western drugs responded to her condition, she came for Tuina treatment.

Physical examination: Slight swelling in the suprolateral condyle of her right elbow, tenderness (+), and tennis elbow test (+).

Diagnosis: External Humeral Epicondylitis on the Right Side.

Cure: After 15 minutes of treatment, her pain was obviously abated. 5 more treatments in succession saw the patient thoroughly recovered. One year later, we made follow-ups and found no recurrence.

2. Periarthritis of Shoulder

Periarthritis of shoulder, also known as omalgia, is mostly seen in people in their fifties, hence also called "fifty-year-old shoulder". For the patient who suffers from protracted motor impairment in the shoulder joint, it is called "congealed shoulder" in ancient Chinese medicine.

Etiology and Pathogenesis

The main factors for the disease are debility due to senility, Qi and Blood Insufficiency, Deficiency of Liver Yin and Kidney Yin; affection of Pathogenic Wind-Cold-Dampness for long-term residence in a damp circumstance; trauma in the shoulder joint. All the factors mentioned-above may lead to loss of nutrients in muscles and Tendons, and consequently the disease.

Clinical Manifestations

This disease is characterized mainly by pain in the shoulder joint and disturbance of shoulder activities.

At its initial stage, the disease is characterized with paroxysmal pain, then persistent pain which becomes more serious day by day, difficulty lying on the affected side, disturbance of sleep by pain at night, accompanied by aversion to cold, pain in turning the shoulder joint, and extensive tenderness around the diseased locale, which radiates to the neck and elbow.

At the later stage, there appears motor disturbance of the shoulder (difficulty in combing, dressing, washing, or reaching the shoulder with his (her) own hand), disuse myatrophy in the deltoideus and acromion projection, thus the congeal shoulder (Fig. 136).

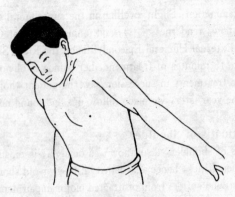

Fig. 136　Congealed Shoulder

Tuina manoeuvres

Principal methods: Treat the disease by Rolling, Kneading with the Palm Base, Kneading-pinching, Dotting with the Flexed Finger, Grasping, Rotating the Shoulder, Abducting the Shoulder, Adducting the Shoulder, Extending and Flexing the Shoulder, Pulling the Shoulder, Rubbing with Both Palms and Shaking.

Subordinate methods: In addition to the tender spots, press and knead Jianyu (LI 15), Tianzong (SI 11), Binao (LI 14), Naoshu (SI 10), Jianjing (GB 21), Quchi (LI 11), and Hegu (LI 4).

Carry out the performance once a day or every other day.

Notes:

In the course of Tuina therapy, it is better for the patient to
do some of the following exercises so as to be recovered as early
as possible.

Climbing the wall: Stand facing a wall. Climb up with both
hands to have the two arms
raised as high as possible, then
put the arms down slowly to
their original position (Fig.
137). Repeat the actions again
and again.

Bending the waist and rotate
the shoulder: Extend the arms
and bend the waist. Move the

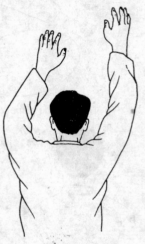

Fig. 137 Climbing the Wall

diseased arm round and round clockwise and anticlockwise 10 — 20 times. The action scope should be gradually increased (Fig. 138). It is better to be done 3—4 times a day.

Dragging the hand on the waist: Put both hands on the lumbar re-gion. Drag the wrist of the diseased side with the healthy hand, then lift it upwards gradually (Fig. 139). Repeat it 3 times a day.

Swinging the arms: The patient stands steadily. Swing both arms backwards and forwards with flexion and extension of the shoulders (Fig. 140), then abduct and adduct both shoulder joints again and again (Fig. 141). The manipulation scope should be from small to large. Repeat it 3—4 times a day.

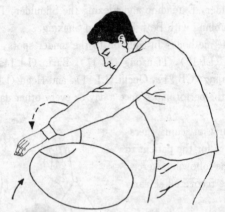

Fig. 138 Bending the Waist and Rock the Shoulder

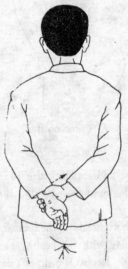

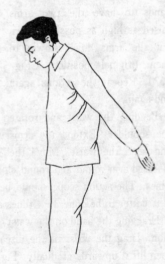

Fig. 139 Dragging the   Fig. 140 Swinging the Arms(1)
Hand on the Waist

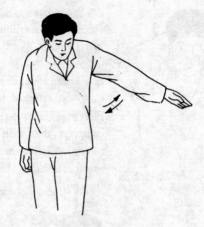

Fig. 141　Swinging the Arms（2）

Everting the arms: Lean against the wall. Clench the hands to make void fists, flex the arms, then evert the arms with the dorsa of hands touching the wall (Fig. 142).

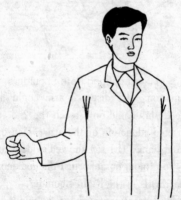

Fig. 142　Everting the Arm

Adducting and abduction both shoulders: Put the crossed two hands on the nape. Adduct both shoulders (Fig. 143) and then abduct them(Fig. 144) to the largest degree.

Case

Qu, female, 53, cadre. First visit: May 8, 1986.

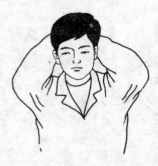

Fig. 143 Adducting Both Shoulders

Symptoms: Pain in the right shoulder joint with motor disturbance for a month.

Case history: The onset of the disease began a month ago, since the patient was attacked by cold at night. She once accept treatment of hot compress, but with little help. Recently her condition became more serious. Therefore she came for Tuina therapy.

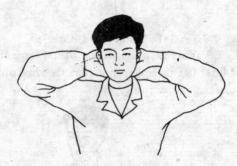

Fig. 144 Abducting Both Shoulders

Physical examination: Her diseased arm could lift to 80° and abduct to 30°; the thumb could only reach the 2nd spinous process owing to the restricted adduction of the arm; Tianzong (SI 11) on the diseased side and Jianyu (LI 15) showed evident tenderness; and the X-ray examination found no abnormal phenomenon.

Diagnosis: Periarthritis in the Right Shoulder.

Cure: Treated by 1 treatment (about 20 minutes), the patient perceived great alleviation of the pain. After 6 treatments, all her symptoms disappeared. Eight years of follow-ups found no recurrence.

3. Injury of Wrist Joint

Wrist joint get injured easily owing to its frequency use every day. If it can not be treated properly or in time, chronic strain in the diseased portion will be formed.

Etiology and Pathogenesis

The disease is often caused by fall, stumble, trauma, or strain and contusion, which lead to inflammatory changes of the soft tissues (muscles, tendons, ligaments, and tendon sheath)around the affected wrist. Finally, there will appear swelling, hyperplasia, adhesion, even motor impairment in the wrist joint.

Clinical Manifestations

The disease is manifested by local swelling, distension, obvious tenderness, and also pain, which is aggravated when the wrist is flexed or extended. If the pain occurs at the styloid process of the radius when the wrist flexes towards the ulnar side, the injury is associated the radial collateral ligament; otherwise, with the ulnar collateral ligament. If the pain appears when the wrist flexes toward the dorsal side, the injury is related to the dorsal carpal ligament and extensor muscle; otherwise, to the palmar ligament and flexor muscle. When the pain occurs as the wrist turns to any direction, in combination with obvious motor impairment, the injury is associated with both ligaments and muscles.

Tuina manoeuvres

Principal methods: Treat the disease by Kneading with the Finger, Rolling, Pressing, Grasping, Pulling the Wrist, Rotating the Wrist and Straight-rubbing.

Subordinate methods: Knead the tender spots, Yangchi (SJ 4), Yangxi (LI 5), Lieque (LU 7), Daling (PC 7), Shaohai (HT 3).

The treatment should be given once a day or every other day.

Case

Xu, male, 39, worker. First visit: June 9, 1992.

Symptoms: Traumatic injury in the wrist for a day.

Case history: The patient got his right wrist sprained when falling from his bike yesterday. He felt painful in the wrist and could not move it.

Physical examination: There was slight swelling at the radial aspect and evident tenderness; the pain was aggravated when the wrist was flexed towards the ulnar side; and the X-ray examination was normal.

Diagnosis: Sprain of the Radial Collateral Ligament.

Cure: Treated with the therapies mentioned-above only for once (15 minutes), the patient had his pain alleviated instantly. After 6 successive treatments, his pain basically disappeared; there was no tenderness on the locale; and the wrist joint restored to its original functions. Three months of follow-ups found no recurrences after the patient was discharged.

4. Injury of Finger Joint

Etiology and Pathogenesis

Of all the types of this disease, injuries of the collateral ligaments and articular capsule in the interphalangeal joint are mostly seen a-mong the patients. The direct factors for the disease are external brutal forces, which result in laceration of the tendon collaterals, and trauma of the articular captule, which in turn bring about such pathological changes as bleeding, swelling, and adhesion on the affected locale.

Clinical Manifestations

It is manifested by swelling around the affected joint, tenderness of the tendon collaterals on both sides, and restricted activities of the diseased digital joint. In the case of laceration of the tendon collaterals, there will appear local deformity, inclination of the digital joint to the affected side.

Tuina manoeuvres

Principal methods: Use Twisting, Kneading with the Finger, Pressing, Pulling the Finger, Rotating the Finger and Regulating.

Subordinate Therapies Press and knead the tender spots, Waiguan (SJ 5), and Jianjing (GB 21).

Carry out the performance once a day or every other day.

Case

Hou, male, 28. First visit: Feb. 26, 1989.

Symptoms: Injury of the middle finger for 3 days.

Case history: The patient had the first segment of his middle finger injured 3 days ago when playing volleyball. After that, there appeared swelling and difficulty of movement on the locale. The patient was subjected to some medicated plaster and washing with Chinese medicine, but his condition did not take a turn for the better. So he came here to adopt Tuina therapies.

Physical examination: There showed sensitive tenderness, debility in flexion and extension of the affected finger, and also severe swelling in the first segment of the diseased finger, which was spindle-shaped. The X-ray examination revealed no abnormal phenomenon.

Diagnosis: Injury of the Middle Finger Joint.

Using the Tuina methods for 15 minutes, we found that the diseased finger was more flexible (30°), and the pain assuaged. After 10 treatments, the pain on the locale disappeared, with tenderness (–), and flexion to 80°. One month later, he was completely recovered and able to work as usual.

5. Tendosynovitis of Styloid Process of Radius

Etiology and Pathogenesis

Tendon sheath, which plays the role of protecting the synovial bursa of muscle tendon, is composed of two layers: the internal and the external. The former attaches tightly to the tendon muscle, and is separated from the external layer through the synovial cavity, which can reduce the friction of muscle tendons by synovial fluid (Fig. 145). Long-term overwork, repeated trauma in the thumb,

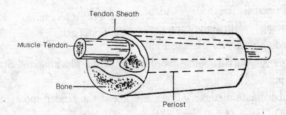

Fig. 145 Model of Tendon Sheath

and attack of Cold pathogens may all result in traumatic inflammation of the tendon sheath, which contains the long abductor muscle and short extensor muscle of the thumb (Fig. 146). It may even lead to edema, thickening of the tendon sheath and adhesion in the

97

affected area. As time goes on, the tendon sheath will constrict and nodules will occur.

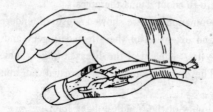

Fig. 146 Tendon Sheath of Radial Styloid Process

Clinical Manifestation

The disease is commonly manifested by sudden pain at the styloid process of the radius, which radiates to the hand, arm, and even shoulder, and is aggravated when the wrist or the thumb is in use. The other symptoms and signs are debility and restricted abducent movement of the affected thumb. There are nodular masses and sensitive tenderness on the diseased locale. Pain occurs when the patient clenches his (her) hand to its ulnar side (Fig. 147). The X-ray examination shows normal results.

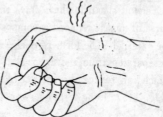

Fig. 147 Clenching the Fist Test

Tuina manoeuvres

Principal methods: Adopt Kneading with the Finger, Kneading with the Thenar Eminence, Rolling, Rubbing-kneading, Rubbing-plucking and Straight-rubbing.

Subordinate methods: Press and knead the tender spots, Yangxi (LI 5), Hegu (LI 4), and Shousanli (LI 10).

The treatment should be performed once a day or every other day.

6. Thecal Cyst

Etiology and Pathogenesis

Thecal Cyst commonly occurs at the dorsal wrist, the lateral side of the wrist and palm, the dorsa of hand or foot, lateral aspect of the knee, and popliteal fossa. It is mostly seen among youths and the middle-aged , especially among women. The causes which lead to the disease are not clear yet. However, it is found in clinical practice that this disease is closely related to trauma.

Clinical Manifestations

Commonly thecal cyst occurs gradually. The nodule, which grows slowly, is smooth on surface, sometimes movable, or changeable in its circumference. There is a local soreness and pain radiating towards the tissues around. When the cysts and the tendon sheath are connected, there will appear flaccidity and debility in the farther extremities.

Tuina manoeuvres

Principal methods: Use Pressing, Rubbing-Plucking, Kneading with the Finger, Pushing, and Straight-rubbing.

Subordinate methods: In addition to the tender spots, press and knead the local points and points on the corresponding Channels.

Case

Xu, female, 25, cadre. First visit: Oct. 6, 1982.

Symptoms: A mass on the right foot dorsum for 2 years.

Case history: Two years ago, there appeared a nodular mass on the dorsum of her right foot and sometimes she perceives a sore and distending sensation around the spot. As time went on, the nodular mass became larger, accompanied by locale soreness and pain especially after a long walk.

Physical examination: There was a nodular mass about 2.5 x 2.5 cm and slight tenderness on the locale. When pressed, the mass would slip upwards or downwards. Its surface is normal. The activities of the ankle and the metatarsophalangeal joints were also normal.

Diagnosis: Thecal Cyst on the Right Foot Dorsum.

Cure: First, we kneaded the diseased part with the thumb belly for 0.5—1 minute, then pressed the nodular mass briskly, quickly and strenuously. A fizzing sound was heard during the operation.

At last, we plucked the nodular mass for 3—5 times and pushed and kneaded the diseased areas for 2—3 minutes. The patient was radically recovered after Tuina treatment. Twelve years of follow-ups found no recurrence.

7. Shoulder-hand Syndrome

Etiology and Pathogenesis

. Shoulder-hand Syndrome refers to the disease marked by pain and rigidity of the shoulder region in combination with swelling, distention, and pain of the hand on the affected side.

Etiology and Pathogenesis

The disease is caused mostly by such pathological changes as retrogressive changes in cervical vertebra, trauma in the neck and shoulder, cerebrovascular or pulmonary diseases, cardiac infarction, etc., which lead to vegetative nerve functional disturbance, dystrophy of vascular nerves in the shoulder and hand.

Clinical Manifestations

This disease is commonly encountered among the old or middle-aged people. It is manifested by pain, usually dull or burning pain in its severe case, consequently stiffness of the digital and wrist joints, swelling and distention of the hand, with tight, shiny, grey-colored skin and low temperature. With the progression of the disease, there occurs gradual muscle atrophy, Dupuytren's contracture, which lead to stiff and deformed joints. The symptoms may be gradually remitted several months later after the onset. Some patients may get some sequels like motor impairment in the hand and shoulder and others.

Tuina manoeuvres

Principal methods: Treat the disease by Rolling, Kneading with the Finger, Kneading with the Palm-base, Grasping, Kneading-pinching, Pressing, Rotating, Twisting, Regulating, Shaking, Rubbing with Both Palms and Rubbing with Both Thenar Eminences.

Subordinate methods: Press and knead Jianyu (LI 15), Jianjing (GB 21), Bingfeng (SI 12), Tianzong (SI 11), Binao (LI 14), Quyuan (SI 13), Quchi (LI 11), Shousanli (SI 10), Hegu (LI 4).

The performance should be given once a day or once two days.

Case

Hu, male, 52, cadre. First visit: March 6, 1989.

Symptoms: Pain and rigidity in the left shoulder for 15 days accompanied with swelling of the hand on the same side.

Case history: Half a month ago, the patient felt stiff in his left shoulder and difficult to raise it for no reasons. There also occurred swelling and distention of the hand on the affected side. He once took medicine like indomethacin and adopted medicated plaster around the locale, but without any effects. So he came for Tuina treatment.

Physical examination: The surface of the diseased shoulder was normal; there was tenderness in Tianzong (SI 11), and Shousanli (LI 10); the arm could only lift at 120° and abduct at 60°; there appeared swelling and disturbance in flexion and extention of the index and middle finger with tight and shiny skin and purplish color, and also low-grade muscular atrophy at the thenar eminence and dorsum of the hand. At the same time, the assay of blood sedimentation, mucin, and blood examination are all normal. The X-ray examination revealed straightness of the physiological curvature in the cervical vertebrae, hyperosteogeny at the anterior margins of the 4th, 5th, and 6th cervical vertebrae, and normal intervertebral spaces.

Diagnosis: Shoulder-hand Syndrome on the Left Side.

Cure: Treated by the above-mentioned manoeuvres for the disease only once (about 20 minutes), the patient felt his symptoms remarkably alleviated. Six Tuina treatments cured him of his disease completely. One year of follow-ups found no recurrence of his morbid state.

Injury of Neck

1. Sprain and Contusion of Neck

Etiology and Pathogenesis

This disease is mostly caused by over-flexion, over-extension and over-rotation of the neck out of carelessness, which result in the Qi

Stagnation and Blood Stasis, hence obstruction in the Channels and Collaterals around.

Clinical Manifestations

The morbid condition is marked by pain in the affected area and restricted movement in the cervical vertebrae, muscular and ligmental spasm, swelling, and obvious tenderness around the diseased part. The pain is usually aggravated in the movement of the cervical vertebrae. The X-ray examination is normal.

Tuina Manoeuvres

Principal methods: Use Rolling, Kneading with the Palm Base, Kneading with the Finger, Pressing, Grasping, Pulling the Neck Semi-circularly, Rotating the Neck and Opening-shutting-rubbing.

Subordinate methods: Grasp Jianjing (GB 21), and knead Tian-zong(SI 11), Dazhui (DU 14), and Hegu (LI 4).

Perform the operation everyday or every other day.

2. Cervical Spondylopathy

Etiology and Pathogenesis

Cervical spondylopathy results mostly from pathological changes such as hyerplasia in the cervical vertebrae and retrograde degeneration of their intervertebral disks, which bring stimulation or oppression on the nerve root, vertebral artery, spinal cord or the sympathetic nerve. Senility, general asthenia, acute or chronic trauma, or attack of Wind-Cold-Dampness lead to the disease more easily. Most of the patients are over the middle-aged, and it is found clinically that the incidence is 100% in people above the age of seventy.

Clinical Manifestations

According to its different symptoms and signs, cervical spondylopathy can be classified into the following types:

Nerve-root type: Manifested by pain accompanied by radiating pain on one side or both sides of the shoulder, heaviness and debility of the upper limbs, cold extremities, and motor impairment in the cervical vertebrae, all of which are shown positive through the squeeze test of intervertebral foramens (Fig. 148) and the stretch test of brachial plexus nerves (Fig. 149).

Vertebral-artery type: Marked by dizziness, migraine, nausea,

102

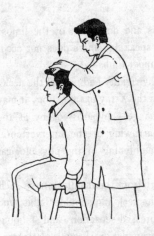

Fig. 148 Intervertebral Foramen Squeeze Test

vomiting, blurred vision, tinnitus, deafness, cervico-occipital pain or pain in the neck and shoulder, and occasional cataplexy. The test of rotating the neck is positive.

Spinal-cord type: Characterized by numbness, soreness, unilateral or bilateral flaccidity of the extremities, spasmodic neck and shoulder, spasmodic paralysis such as difficulty in movement, staggering or unsteady walk, hypermyotonia, tendon hyperreflexia, attenuation or disappearance of superficial reflex, and other pathological reflexes involving sensory and motor impairment.

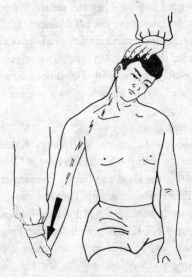

Fig. 149 Brachial Plexus Stretch Test

Sympathetic-nerve type: Marked by occipital pain, palpitation, oppressed feeling in the chest, cold limbs and skin, burning sensa-

103

tion of the hand and foot, soreness and distention of the limbs, headache, dizziness, etc. Generally speaking, there does not occur radiating pain and numbness in the upper limbs.

Neck (cervical) type: Manifested by rigidity and pain of the neck, and disturbance in its movement. On the X-ray examination, it may found the following pathological changes: hyperosteogeny at the margins of the vertebral body , narrowing of the intervertebral spaces, ligamental calcification, straightening of the physiological curvature, etc.

Coronary-heart-disease type: Apart from the manifestations such as soreness and pain and malaise in the neck and shoulder, this type of disease is marked by tight and oppressed sensation, and stabbing pain in the precordial regions. The examination through electrocardiogram finds no abnormal results.

Deglutive-disturbance type: Marked by foreign-body sensation in the throat when swallowing and dysphagia with progressive improvement, alleviated or gone when the patient bends forwards and aggravated when he (she) raise the head backwards. The X-ray examination shows that there occur pathological spurs along the anterior border between the 5th and 6th cervical vertebrae in most of the patients, thus resulting in the morbid conditions mentioned-above.

Complexed (mixed) type: Marked by two or more types of symptoms mentioned-above.

Tuina manoeuvres

Principal methods: Manipulate by Rolling, Kneading with the Palm Base, Kneading with the Finger, Pressing, Grasping, Pulling up the Neck, Lifting the Head and Neck, Pinching-grasping, Rubbing with Both Palms, Rubbing with Thenar Eminences, Shaking, When the patient feels headache, add Pushing-wiping, Pushing the Forehead Divergently and Grasping with the Five Fingers.

Subordinate methods: In addition to the tender spots, press and knead the following points: Jianzhongshu (SI 15), Jianwaishu (SI 14), Jianjing (GB 21), Fengmen (BL 12), Jianyu (LI 15), Quchi (LI 11), Shousanli (SI 10), Hegu(LI 4), Xiaohai (ST18), Neiguan (PC 60, Waiguan(SJ 5). Add the kneading of Taiyang (Ex−HN),

Jingming (BL 1), Yuyao (Ex−HN), Tinggong (SI 19), and Baihui (DU 20) to the patient who suffers from headache.

Perform the operation everyday or every other day.

Case 1

Zhang, male, 50. First visit: Feb. 15, 1990.

Symptoms: Pain in the back and shoulder for 6 months accompanied with numbness and soreness and pain of the right limb.

Case history: The patient was chilled half a year ago, thus resulting in pain in the neck and shoulder regions, accompanied by pain and numbness of the upper limb. In the recent days, his conditions turned worse and worse. A large quantity of Chinese and western drugs failed to make improvement. Therefore, he came to receive Tuina treatment.

Physical examination: There existed rigidity in the cervical vertebrae, tenderness on the area between the 5th and 6th vertebrae and at Tianzong (SI 11) of the diseased side, positive reflexes both in the squeezing test of the intervertebral foramens and the tug test of the brachial plexus nerves. The X-ray examination showed that there occurred straightening of the physiological curvature in the cervical vertebrae, hypermyotonia at the anterior margins of the 5th, 6th, and 7th cervical vertebrae, slight narrowing in their spaces, and calcification of the longitudinal ligaments.

Diagnosis: Cervical Spondylopathy of Nerve-root Type.

Cure: By the manipulations mentioned above for one time (about 20 minutes), the patient felt much better. After 6 treatments in succession, the painful and numb sensation in the upper limbs on the neck and back vanished. Then 4 more treatments, his illness was completely cured. Two years of follow-ups found no recurrence.

Case 2

Chai, female, 40. First visit: March 6, 1987.

Symptoms: Vertigo, migraine, soreness and pain in the neck, nausea, vomiting and malaise in the neck.

Case history: She got the symptoms above a year ago. She once accepted treatment in another hospital and was admitted to take Chinese and western drugs like theohydramine, VitB6, pills for refreshment of the brain, etc., but failed to have obvious effects. In the last several months, her state became more and more serious, complicated by blurred vision, dryness of the eyes, tinnitus and aggravation of dizziness in head turning and head raising.

Physical examination: It was found that the patient's muscles in the neck were tense and rigid; she felt dizzy and tended to vomit when lifting up the head because of the blurred vision. Her blood pressure was 16/10.7 kPa. The X-ray examination revealed such pathological changes as sharpening of the 4th, 5th, and 6th vertebral articulations, low-grade hyperplasia at the posterior margins of the 5th and 6th cervical vertebrae, narrowing of their interspaces, and straightening in their physiological curvature. The report of rheoencephalogram showed that the vertebrobasilar arterial blood vessel was in a contractive state, thus resulting in decrease of blood supplication.

Diagnosis: Cervical Spondylopathy of Vertebral-artery Type.

Cure: According to the pathologic changes and manifestations of the patient, we adopted the following manipulations: first, operate on the head by Pushing-wiping, Pushing the Forehead Divergently, Kneading with the Finger, and Grasping with the Five Fingers (put the left hand on the patient's forehead to fix it, apply strength through the five branched-out fingers and grasp the head from the anterior hairline to the occipital part for 10 times (Fig. 150); then on the neck and back by Rolling, Kneading with the Palm Base, Grasping, and Pulling up the Neck. In addition, press and knead Taiyang (Ex — HN), Zanzhu (BL 2), Jingming (BL 1), Yuyao (Ex — HN), Tinggong (SI 19), Baihui (DU 20), Fengchi (GB 20), Fengfu

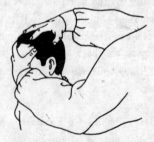

Fig. 150 Grasping with the Five Fingers

(DU 16), Jianjing (GB 21), Tianzong(SI 11), and Shousanli (SI 10).

After 1 treatment by the manoeuvres mentioned-above (20 minutes or so), her symptoms like dizziness were immediately alleviated. Three times more found vertigo, migraine and cervico-occipital pain strikingly assuaged, and blurred vision relieved. Six times later, all her morbid conditions disappeared. The re-examination of rheoencephalogram showed normal results. Ever since she was discharged, no recurrence was found.

3. Stiff-neck

This disease refers to pain, stiffness, soreness, distention, myospasm and motor disturbance of the neck. It may be a premonitory symptom of cervical spondylopathy among the adults. The patient whose condition is mild can be recovered in several days, the one whose condition is serious may be affected by it for many weeks. Tuina therapy is very effective for the disease.

Etiology and Pathogenesis

It is mostly caused by overfatigue, uncomfortable pillow, improper lying posture, attack of wind and cold, sudden turning the neck, or overloading on one side of the shoulders, leading to myospam of the neck, dislocation of the cervical intervertebral articulations, or incarceration of the articular synovium, thus the disease.

Clinical Manifestations

The manifestations of the disease are pain, rigidity and spasm of the sternocleidomastoid muscle on one side or both sides of the neck, which may radiate to the trapezius and levator muscle of the scapula. The patient tends to incline his (her) head to the diseased side, and the mandible to the healthy side. It is obvious that the patient' neck is restricted in its movement, especially when it turns to the diseased side. The pain may even involve the head, upper limbs and upper back. There occur muscular tension, and sensitive tenderness, and may also occur local tender spots on both sides of the spinous process.

Tuina manoeuvres

Principal methods: Use Rolling on the Back (Fig. 151), Knead-

ing with the Palm Base, Grasping, Pulling the Neck Semi-circularly, Rotating the Neck as well as Opening-shutting-rubbing.

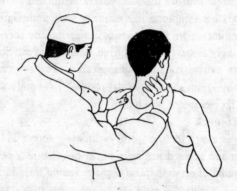

Fig. 151   Rolling on the Back

Subordinate methods: Press and knead Fengchi (G2), Fengfu
(DU 16), Fengmen (BL 12), Tianzong (SI 11), and Jianjing (GB
21).

Perform the manipulations once a day for 3 days in succession.

Case

Zhao, female, 32, cadre. First visit: Oct. 25, 1989.

Symptoms: Stiffness and pain, with motor impediment of the
neck for 1 day.

Case history: The patient found her neck painful, stiff and difficulty in turning when getting up in the morning. She attached some
medicated plaster on the locale, but with little help. Instead, her
condition became more serious. So, she came for Tuina treatment.

Physical examination: The cervical vertebrae of the patient tended
to incline to the left anterior side; the trapezius muscle was tense;
there was evident tendeness by the 5th and 6th vertebrae and at the
point of Tianzong (SI 11).

Diagnosis: Stiff-neck.

Cure: Just treated for ten minutes by the manipulations mentioned-above, the patient had her symptoms alleviated and relieved.
She was completely cured of her illness the next day.

108

Injury of Waist and Back

1. Prolapse of Lumbar Intervertebral Disc

Prolapse of the intervertebral disc is one of the main reasons causing sciatic nerve pain. It is often seen in people aging from 20—45, who are engaged in physical labour. The patient usually suffers from sharp pain and is susceptible to be seized with chronic lumbocrual pain. With Tuina therapy, the effective rate of 95%—100% and cure rate of 71%—87% can be achieved.

Etiology and Pathogenesis

Traumatic and Accumulative Strain: Lumbar sprain and accumulative strain are main reasons causing damage of the fibrous rings. The lumbar vertebrae sticks out anteriorly when the intervertebral disc is thin in the rear and thick in the front. When propel bend over, the pulpiform nucleus moves to the rear and produces great elasticity under the tension force of the body weight, muscle and ligament, whose force is in proportion with the pressure of weight that it carries. When the force is too strong or the fibrous rings of the intervertebral disc have defects, the pulpiform nucleus may break the fibrous rings and sticks out to the rear and causes pressure on the nerve root, cauda equima and spinal cord (Fig. 152).

Physiological Retrogression: With age growing, the fibrous rings lose their original elasticity and water in the pulpiform nucleus diminishes. Due to that reason, the tissue slowly loses its original function and the fibrous rings become thinner and thinner until rupture occurs under repetitious pressure, thus the pulpiform nucleus may stick out from the broken part.

Pathogenic Cold and Emotional factors: Some patients have no trauma or strain, however, lumbar and back muscle may have spasm when the body catches cold or being emotionally stimulated. The small blood vessel shrinks when chilled, causing ineffective blood circulation and poor intervertebral disc nutrition. Besides, the muscle spasm increases the pressure on the intervertebral disc, which further hurts the intervertebral disc that has expanded (Fig.

109

153), thus the pulpiform nucleus sticks out.

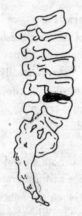 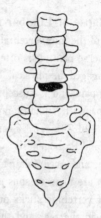

Fig. 152　Pulpiform Nucleus　Fig. 153　Expansion of Lumbar
Protruding Backward　　　　　Intervertebral Disc

In addition, immunology holds that pulpiform nucleus is certain substance that does not relate to blood cycling, thus autoimmune mechanism have no influence on it. When the fibrous rings and lamina cartilage plate are injured and disruptive, the contact with the granulation tissues with no blood will cause retrogression and rupture in pulpiform nucleus.

Clinical Manifestations

Lumbago and sciatica: Pain is often felt in waist region first, then lower limbs, aggravated when the patient coughs, sneezes or defecates forcefully. The patients can hardly bend over and squat down, some can even not take care of himself. Scoliosis: Most patients have their spinal column twisted to various extent. The direction of the side flange shows the position of the projection and its relation with the nerve. If the pulpiform nucleus sticks out from posterolateral and presses the anterior medial part of the nerve root, the spinal column bends towards the affected part and sticks out to the healthy part (Fig. 154). If the pulpiform nucleus sticks out from the posterolateral side and oppresses the anterolateral nerve root, the spinal column will bend towards the healthy side and sticks out

110

to the affected side (Fig. 155).

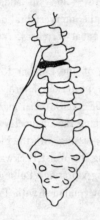 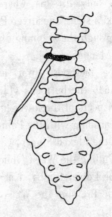

Fig. 154 Lumbar Intervertebral Disc Oppressing the Anteriormedial Aspect or the Nerve Root of the Nerve Root

Fig. 155 Lumbar Intervertebral Disc Oppressing the Anterolateral Aspect of the Nerve Root

Tenderness: Pathological changes occur at the spot 1—2 cm lateral to the spinous process of the lumbar vertebrae, with pain and radiating pain in the farther lower extremities, and tenderness at the following acupoints: Juliao (GB 29), Huantiao (GB 30), Weizhong (BL 40), Yanglingquan (GB 34) and Juegu (GB 39). The protrusion of the 4th and 5th lumbar intervertebral disc may constrict the 5th lumbar nerve root, so pain radiates from the buttocks to the big toe, via the posterior aspect of the thigh and lateral aspect of the shank. If protrusion occurs at the 1st vertebral disk of the 5th sacrum, the nerve root of the 1st sacrum will be oppressed and the pain would radiate from the lumbosacral portion to the little toe, via the posterior aspect of the lower limb and the sole. If the protrusion locates at the centre or moves within the vertebral canal, there may occur radiating pain in the lower limbs and even worse, involuntary discharge of urine may happen. If protrusion occurs between the 1st and 3rd lumbar vertebrae, radiating pain of the femoral nerve will appear.

The leg-straightened lifting test shows that the patient in a severe case can only lift his (her) legs to 15°— 30°. In addition, Brudzinski's sign is positive. Protrusion of the intervertebral disc is visible through the scanning of CT in the lumbar vertebrea.

Tuina Manouevres

Principal methods: First, adopt Rolling on the Lumbar Region (Fig. 156), the buttocks (Fig. 157), the posterior, lateral, and anterior aspects of the lower limbs (Fig. 158—160); then, manipulate by Kneading with the Palm Base, Dredging the Channels, Dotting with the Flexed Finger, Grasping, Suppressing with the Flexed Elbow, Pulling the Waist Obliquely, Pulling the Waist Backwards, Lifting the Lower Limbs, Kneading-pressing-vibrating, Pulling the Legs while Pressing the Waist, Pushing, or combined with Trampling.

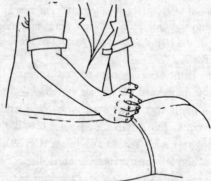

Fig. 156   Rolling on the Lumbar Region

Subordinate methods: In addition to the tender spots, press and knead Juliao (GB 29), Huantiao (GB 30), Chengfu (BL 36), Yinmen (BL 37), Weizhong (BL 40), Yanglingquan (GB 34), Xuanzhong (GB 39), and Kunlun (BL 60).

Perform the operations once a day for 12 times in succession as a course of treatment.

Case

Wang, male, 45, first visit: Aug. 17, 1991.

Symptoms: Pain in the waist and left-lower limb for more than 3

112

months.

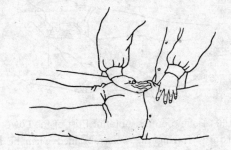

Fig. 157   Rolling on the Buttocks

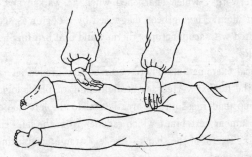

Fig. 158   Rolling on the Posterior Part of the Lower Limbs

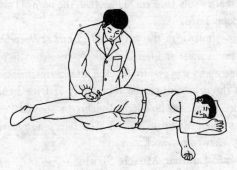

Fig. 159   Rolling on the Lateral Part of the Lower Limbs

113

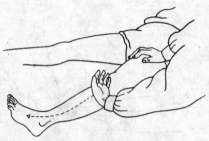

Fig. 160   Rolling on the Anterior Part of the Lower Limbs

Case history: Having the waist sprained when he lifted heavy things in May 1991. He suffered from lumbago and had lumbocrural pain afterwards, which sharpened when he walked and was even worse at night. Having been diagnosed by a doctor as sciatica pain and treated with acupuncture, therapy and oral bruffin, he still suffered a lot.

Physical examination: There occurred low-graded lateral inclination of the lumbar vertebrae, straightening of physiological curvature, deep tenderness on the area lateral to the left side of the 4th and 5th lumbar vertebrae, which radiates from the left sciatic nerve area to the lateral of the shank. The leg-straightened lifting test and the neck-curving test showed positive. The CT scanning of the lumbar vertebrae revealed that the 4th and 5th intervertebral disc protruded left-backwards (0.5 cm higher than the normal) and the dura mater was oppressed.

Diagnosis: Prolapse of the 4th and 5th Lumbar Vertebrae.

Cure: Pain in waist and left lower limb was instantly relieved after 1 treatment and was greatly relieved after 3 treatments. After 10 treatments the pain disappeared thoroughly and the lumbar vertebrae resumed its normal function. Tenderness showed (−) and the lower limbs could lift up to 90°. A year later, he recovered completely and renewed his work.

2. Chronic Lumbar Muscle Strain

The chronic lumbar muscle strain means prolonged injury of the soft tissues such as lumbosacral portion and fascia, etc.

Etiology and Pathogenesis

If untreated promptly and thoroughly and taking place repeatedly, the acute injury to the ligaments and muscles in the waist may result in local blood oozing, fibrous degeneration and the appearance of sear tissue, which oppresses or stimulate the nerve and leads to chronic lumbago. People who often carry heavy objects on one shoulder, bend the waist and get habitual abnormal posture usually get lumbar and spinal soreness as a result of overfatigue. Some patient get diseased owing to congenital deformity, such as unilateral sacralization or asymmetrical minor intervertebral joints, which leads to disturbance of activities on the sides of the lumbosacral portion.

Clinical Manifestations

Lumbago reoccurs often in those who get a long term case history. Soreness is felt on one of both sides of the lumbosacral portion, usually alleviated after rest and work; pain is felt extensively in the deceased part when pressed yet tenderness is not evident; no severe meonuenience is perceived in the lower limbs. When the disease is severe, muscular spasm, lateral curvature of the spinal column and pain in lower limbs may occur. For those who get rheumatism, pachylosis and insensitivity is perceived in the diseased part.

Tuina Manouevres

Principal methods: Adopt Rolling, Kneading with the Palm Base, Pressing, Tapping and Straight-rubbing with the Polythenar Eminences on the lumbosacral portion and either side of the Bladder Channel.

Subordinate methods: Press and knead Shenshu (BL 23), Eight-liaos, Weizhong (BL 40), and the tender spots.

The treatment should be given once a day or every other day.

Notes

The patients need to correct timely their habitual abnormal posture and enhance the muscular functions of the loins and back (Fig. 161). It is better to use hard-board bed and try to warm the lumbar region and alleviate the weight the waist has to carry.

115

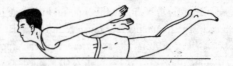

Fig. 161   Enhancing Muscular Functions
of the Loins and Back

Case

Cai, male, 38, worker. First visit: July 16th, 1987.

Symptoms: Lumbago, lasting for more than one year, aggravated for half a month before he came to me.

Case history: The patient got his waist injured a year ago and was seized with lumbago ever since. No curative effect was perceived after taking some medicine. Ever since then, the disease occurred 5 — 6 times every year in case of fatigue or chill. Half a month earlier he felt pain in the waist due to sleeping in the night outside. The pain was aggravated the next morning, which made turning over difficult and limited the squatting and standing of the body. No radiating pain was felt in the lower limbs. Having failed in the treatment with acupuncture and physiotherapy, the patient came for help.

Physical Examination: The physiological curvature of the lumbar vertebrae tends to be straightened; the lumbar vertebrae bended 50° forwards and extended 10° backwards. The leg-straightened lifting test shows (—); no abnormal phenomenon is visible on X-ray examination; blood sedimentation and determination of muscin is normal.

Diagnosis: Chronic Lumbar Muscle Strain.

Cure: Having been treated for 15 minutes with the Tuina method mentioned-above, the pain in the waist was immediately relieved and the lumbar could be straightened. After a repeated treatment , the lumbar pain was greatly alleviated and the lumbar vertebra renewed its normal work. Having got the treatment for a third time in the next day, the lumbago disappeared totally and lumbar vertebrae worked flexibly. The disease did not reoccur .

3. Synovial Incarceration of Posterior Joints of Lumbar Vertebrae

116

This disease is often caused by acute lumbago resulting from sudden change in the position of the posterior joints of the lumbar vertebrae.

Etiology and Pathogenesis

People often get their waist sprained due to abnormal posture of the small joint of the lumbar vertebrae when they bend down or carry heavy things, which , always leads to synovial incarceration of posterior joints of the lumbar vertebrae and the dynamic balance of the spinal column and the coordination function of the spinal are destroyed. Pain and spasm is also perceived at the same time. Inflammatory reactions can be brought about due to synovium incarceration between articular surfaces, which, often results in adhesion of the small joints.

Clinical Manifestation

Stabbing pain is felt shortly after the sprain and the lumbar vertebrae is perceived to be protruding backwards. Spasm is felt in the loins and killing pain appears when people move their lower limbs. Abnormality of the spinous processes may be found by digital palpation. There also appears deep tenderness by the 4th, and 5th lumbar vertebrea, with no radiating pain on the lower extremities.

Tuina Manouevres

Principal methods: Use Rolling, Kneading with the Palm Base, Pressing, Pulling the Waist Semi-circularly, Pulling the Waist Obliquely and Pulling-jerking.

Subordinate methods: Press and knead Weizhong (BL 40) and Chengshan(BL 57).

Case

Liu, male, 45. First visit: Oct. 6, 1992.

Symptoms: Pain in the lumbar region for 6 hours.

Case history: The patient got his waist sprained when he carried heavy things. Sharp pain was instantly felt and activity of the lumbarvertebra was no longer available. He was carried to the doctor for treatment.

Physical examination: No movement in the waist region was available and killing pain was felt instantly once the lower limbs was

117

moved. Spasm existed in the lumbosacral portion. Tenderness showed (+) in the 4th and 5th spinous process and the 5th spinous process deviated slightly.

Diagnosis: Synovial Incarceration of Posterior Joints of the Lumbar Vertebrae.

Cure: The lumbago was relieved shortly after 1 treatment and the lumbar resumed its normal function , which made the patient able to walk by himself. After 1 more treatment, the symptoms disappeared completely and the patient returned to work. No discomfort was felt in the following 3 months.

4. Acute Lumbar Muscle Sprain

The spine column in the lumbar area carries half of the weight of the whole body and takes part in various activities, thus it is prone to be injured.

Etiology and Pathogenesis

This disease usually occurs as a result of incorrect posture in such activities as bending down, carrying heavy objects or being attacked by external force in the waist region. The muscular tissue get acute injury resulting from sharp twist or drug.

Clinical Manifestations

For those who are seriously diseased, sharp pain is felt in the waist and they can not move easily and have difficulty in sitting and lying and turning over, some even can not get up. The pain is aggravated when people coughs or breathes deeply. For those who are slightly diseased, no sharp pain is felt, yet several hours or $1-2$ days later, the pain is aggravated. Usually spasm of greater psoas-muscles on one or both sides appears and most patients feel pressure pain point and the lumbar vertebrae leans towards the diseased part.

Tuina Manouevres

Principal methods: Cure the disease with Rolling, Kneading with the Palm Base, Pressing, Dredging the Channels, Plucking, Straight-rubbing with the Polythenar Eminences.

Subordinate methods: Apart from tender spots, press and knead Shenshu (BL 23), Yaoyangguan (DU 3), and Weizhong (BL 40).

Perform Tuina therapy once a day for 3 days in succession.

118

Case

Liu, male, 24. First visit: May 10th, 1988.

Case history: The patient hurt his waist by carelessness 2 days ago when he was bending down to carry heavy objects before he contracted lumbago. Slight in the day and serious at night, the pain affected his sleep seriously. No effective result having been achieved with treatment such as physiotherapy, he came for help.

Physical examination: the lumbar vertebrae bends to the left and the left psoasmuscle gets slight tumefaction; tenderness was evident; anterior flexion of the lumbar vertebra is 60 and the posterior extension as well as the lateral flexion is 10; no abnormal phenomenon appeared in the anterolateral film of the lumbar vertebrae.

Diagnosis: Left Psoasmusle Sprain.

Cure: Having been treated for 15 minutes with the Tuina method, the lumbago was immediately alleviated and the patient got a sound sleep at night and could turn over flexibly. After 2 treatments the lumbago disappeared and the lumbar vertebrae renewed its normal activity. The patient got thorough recovery 5 months later. No recurrence appeared ever since then.

5. Hypertrophic Spondylitis

Hypertrophic spondylities, also called proliferating spondylities or osteoarthritis spondylitis, is the chronic retrograde degeneration often occurring in the middle-aged or the old people.

Etiology and Pathogenesis

Pathological changes in lumbar intervertebral disc and spongy substance of bones: Intervertebral disc degeneration occurs as people approach their middle ages. The space between the lumbar vertebrae becomes narrow and the elasticity decreases, causing the vertebral ends prone to be vibrated, shocked and worn. Spurs appear as a result of resistance reduction of the lumbar vertebrae due to the substantia spongiosa ossium, which makes the soft tissues nearby oppressed. The spinal cord and the nerve root may be oppressed by the posterior spurs.

Acute and chronic trauma: Frequent sprain and contusion in the waist may results in prolonged aseptic inflammation, and obstruction in Blood circulation, thus leading to inflammatory changes of the articular cartilage and reactionary hyperosteogeny below the cartilage, which often occurs in the young and strong people.

Clinical Manifestations

The principal symptoms and signs are as follows: rigidity, soreness and pain in the waist for sitting over long, in patients over the middle-aged, which are assuaged after some movement but aggravated in the morning and after overwork. Some patients also suffer from numbness, muscular atrophy and even paralysis in the lower limbs. Physical examination shows abnormal physical curvature, local muscle spasm as well as pressure pain. The leg-straightened test reveals a normal condition. Hyperosteogeny is seen on the vertebral border by X-ray examination.

Tuina Manouevres

Principal methods: Use Rolling, Kneading with the Palm Base, Dredging the Channels, Pulling the Waist Obliquely, Rubbing the Lumbosacral Portion with the Palm (Fig. 162), Lifting the Lower Limbs, and Pulling the Waist Backward.

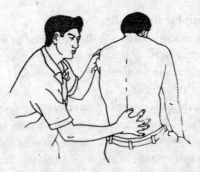

Fig. 162 Rubbing the Lumbosacral
Portion with the Palm

Subordinate methods: Press and knead Mingmen (DU 4), Yaoyangguan (DU 3), Eight-liaos, Weizhong (BL 40), Yanglingquan (GB 34), Chengshan (BL 57).

Case

Ma, female, 53, worker. First visit: Apr. 9th, 1989.

120

Symptoms: Lumbago for more than 2 years; numbness felt for 15 days.

Case history: The patient suffered from lumbago 2 years earlier and felt stiffness in the waist. The condition turned to be worse in the morning. As no effective result had been achieved by acupuncture and oral administration of traditional Chinese medicine and the aggravated lumbago made him too distressed to walk and sleep well, he was accompanied to come for help.

Physical examination: The physiological curvature of the lumbar vertebral straightened; the lumber muscle on both sides tightened; tenderness revealed (+); the lumbar vertebrae curved 40 forward and extended 40 backward. The right lower limb lifted up to 40 while the healthy to 80. The X-ray film showed that biate hyperosteogeny existed in the anterior margin of the 3rd, 4 h and 5th lumbar vertebrae. Hyperosteogeny also existed in the osterior magin of the 5th lumbar vertebra.

Diagnosis: Hypertrophic Spondylitis between the 4th and 5th Lumbar vertebrae.

Cure: After 15 minutes of the treatment as mentioned-above, the lumbago and numbness was instantly relieved and almost disappeared after 6 Tuina treatments. The lumbar vertebra renewed its normal movement and a sound sleep was gained. The patient returned to his routine work after one more week of treatment. The patient was followed up for a year and no recurrence was found.

6. Muscle Strain in Back

Strain of the back muscle is one of the main factors causing back pain, often occurring in the young and strong people.

Etiology and Pathogenesis

For those who take long-term strenuous exercises in their daily work, such as sportsman and fitter, the back muscles, especially those above the trapezius, have long been impaired chronically, which leads to the laceration of the muscle fiber as well as hyperemia and edema.

Clinical Manifestations

Soreness and weakness is felt on one or both sides of the shoulder, which affects the normal movement of the upper limbs. Pain is felt in the spinous process of the back and the internal margin of the scapula , aggravated when the shoulder is in motion. A sense of heaviness is felt in the shoulder and the condition turns to be worse with fatigue, yet alleviated after some movement. Muscle tension exists locally and tenderness shows (+). Some patients have part of the body suffered from chill with weather changes.

Tuina Manouevres

Principal methods: Use Rolling on the Back (Fig. 163), Kneading with the Palm Base, Kneading with the Finger, Grasping, Pressing, Plucking, and Chopping with the Joined Palms.

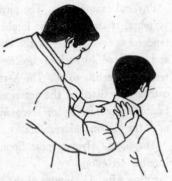

Subordinate methods: In addition to the tender spots, press and knead Jianjing, Bingfeng (SI 12), Quyuan (SI 13,) Jian-waishu (SI 14), Dazhui (DU 14), Naoshu (SI 10), Weizhong (BL 40), Shousanli (LI 10), and Hegu (LI 14).

Fig. 163　Rolling on the Back

Perform the Tuina manoeuvres as mentioned-above once a day or once 2 days.

Case

Chang, male, 30, cadre. First visit: Dec. 6th, 1992.

Symptoms: He suffered from a sore back , accompanied with a sense of heaviness and weakness for more than a year. The disease was aggravated half a month before.

Case history: Long-term hard work which required his hanging head resulted in a sore and powerless back and the pain increased with fatigue and was alleviated after some movement. The condition turned to be worse a month ago because of fatigue and common cold. As no effective result was gained by some treatment as oral in-

122

domethacin and physiotherapy, he came to visit me.

Physical examination: The patient got trapezius muscle tension and tenderness on both shoulders . However, the shoulder joints worked normally and no abnormal phenomenon was revealed in the report of cervical vertebral.

Diagnosis: Muscle Strain on the Back.

Cure: After 20 minutes of 1 Tuina treatment the shoulders were instantly relieved from pain and felt relaxed. At the end of 5 Tuina treatments (1 treatment each day), the symptoms completely disappeared. The patient recovered entirely half a year later and resumed his work. No recurrence had been found ever since then.

7. Tight Chest

The disease of tight chest usually results from Qi Stagnation due to trauma, which brings such symptoms and signs as tight pain, distress and malaise in the chest.

Etiology and Pathogenesis

Inappropriate gesture in daily physical labour often results in traction or oppression of the muscles around the chest, leading to spasm and laceration of the chest wall muscle, internal intercostal muscle, external intercostal muscle, intercostal fascia and anadesma. Together with semiluxation of the costoveretebral joints and synorium incarceration, the intercostal nerves is stimulated and a tight chest is perceived.

Clinical Manifestations

Unfixed pain is instantly felt around the chest and hypotrondrium as a result of trauma. It is aggravated during cough and breath and may radiate to the back, which makes the diseased unable to breathe deeply. For those who got semiluxation in their costovertebral joints, tenderness is felt in part of the body. Swelling and tenderness can be found in the affected locale.

Tuina Manouevres

Principal methods: Use Round-rubbing, Pressing, Kneading, Knocking, Pulling the Shoulder, Extending the Chest, and Straight-rubbing.

Subordinate methods: Press and knead Zhangmen (LIV 13), Qimen (LIV 14), the tender spots and acupoints on the back along the course of the Bladder Channel.

Let the patient sit steadily. First, stroke the diseased part for several minutes first; secondly, dot the corresponding acupoints for 0. 5—1 minute until there appears a local sore, distending sensation, which indicates the arrival of Qi; thirdly, carry out Hugging for one time; fourthly, stretch the shoulder joint by lifting up the patient's arm with the flexed forearm (Fig. 164) so as to regulate the dislocated joint and relieve the spasmodic muscles; finally, ask the patient hold his (her)

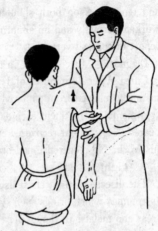

Fig. 164   Tuina Mano-
euvre for Tight Chest (1)

breath, then knock the diseased portion of the patient's back with the palm base of the other hand (Fig. 165—166). Having done all the actions, ask the patient respire deeply .

Carry out the Tuina manipulations once a day or every other day.

8. Sprain of Sacroiliac Joint

The sacroiliac joint locates between the sacrum and the ilium, surrounded by tough ligament to limit its rotation. Sprain of the sacroiliac joint usually results in lumbago.

Etiology and Pathogenesis

Inappropriate movements of the lower limbs, sprain and contusion by external brutal force, or heavy loading and others may lead ad to the injury of the ligaments. On the other hand, affected by endocrine, the female are prone to be injured in their sacroiliac joints during delivery of children, bringing about such asceptic inflammatory reactions as traumatic hyperemia, bleeding, exudation, edema, etc.

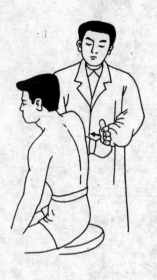 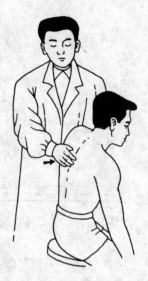

Fig. 165   Tuina Manoeuvre   Fig. 166   Tuina Manoeuvre
        for Tight Chest (2)   for Tight Chest (3)

Clinical Manifestations

Pink bruise and swelling appear around the sacroiliac joint when it is violently attacked. For those who get sprain and contusion owing to falling down, diffuse swelling appears in part of the body and the adhering muscle has spasm , which makes the pelvis of the diseased part incline upwards, thus the diseased leg seems shortened. It is positive in "Figure 4" test (the patient lies down with the healthy leg stretched and the diseased one curved, the diseased foot on the healthy knee, the doctor press the diseased knee with one hand while press the anterior sapercor with another hand to wrench the diseased sacroiliac joint (Fig. 167); it is also positive in the bedside test(Fig 168). (The patient lies down on his back with the diseased hip placed on the bedside. Flex the healthy leg to fix the pelvis. The doctor move the diseased leg on the bedside and extend it backwards to stretch the sacroiliac joint).

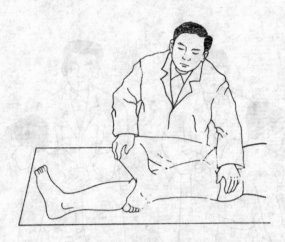

Fig. 167 "Figure 4" Test

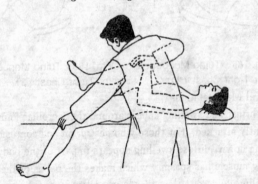

Fig. 168 Bedside Test

Tuina Manouevres

Principal methods: Use Rolling, Kneading with the Palm Base,
Round-rubbing, Pressing, Suppressing with the Flexed Elbow, Ro-
tating the Hip Joint, Straight-rubbing and Revolving with the
Flexed Elbow.

Subordinate methods: Knead and revolve Huantiao (GB 30),
Eight-liaos, and the tender spots.

Carry out the dirigation on the sacro-iliac articulation and its adja-

126

cent tissues of the affected side every day or every other day.

Case

Wang, male, 38, cadre. First visit: Nov. 6th, 1989.

Symptoms: 2 days of lumbago on the left side.

Case history: The patient got his left sacroiliac joint sprained by tumbling carelessly when he rode a bicycle. He could not undertake the regular work because of the lumbago and disability for bending down. Having failed with such treatments as hot conpress and oral administration of Brufen, he came to visit me.

Physical examination: He got slight swelling in the left sacroiliac joint with evident tenderness, and both "Figure 4" test and the bedside test were positive. No abnormal phenomenon was found from the X-ray examination.

Diagnosis: Sprain of the Left Sacroiliac Joint.

Cure: The patient found the pain alleviated instantly after one treatment (15 minutes or so) and almost disappeared after 5 consecutive treatments. Only slight tenderness was felt in part of the body. The "Figure 4" test and bedside test showed (−). With another week of Tuina therapy (1 treatment every other day) totalling 9 times in all, no malaise was felt. The patient recovered completely 3 months later and the disease never recurred ever since then.

Injury of Glutealfemoral Portion

1. Syndrome of M. Pirifomis

The disease refers to a series of pathological changes which take place because of the stenosis of the piriformis out of injuries, spasm and degeneration, which result in stimulation or oppression of the sciatic nerve and other sacral plexus and the buttock blood vessels when passing through the piriform apertura. The disease is one of the factors causing dry sciatic pain.

Etiology and Pathogenesis

The piriformis divides the greater sciatic foramen into two parts: the lower piriform aperture and the upper piriform aperture. In the former, there traverse the sciatic nerve, posterior cutaneous nerve of the thigh, inferior gluteal nerve, pudendal nerve, inferior gluteal artery and vein; and in the latter, there pass the superior gluteal nerve, superior gluteal artery and vein (Fig. 169).

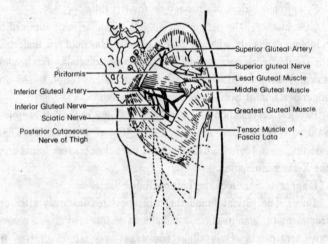

Fig. 169 Nerves and Blood Vessels
Passing through the Upper and
Lower Apertures of the Piriformis

Most patients get their piriformis damaged by sudden extorsion or over-rotation for external forces. Some get the disease when attacked by Wind-Cold-Dampness, resulting in local Blood Stagnation and disturbance of neuroregulation. It is believed by some experts that the syndrome, to some extent, pertains to degeneration of the lumbar vertebrea.

Clinical Manifestations

At the initial stage, dull or stabbing pain is felt by the patient in the buttocks, accompanied by sensation of soreness, swelling, tightening and pain which radiate from the posterolateral shank calf to the dorsum and lateral margin of the foot. There also occur malaise in the perineum and sharp pain in the testis and scrotum, which usually leads to the clumsy walking of the patient. The more serious will be afflicted with unbearable pain in the hip region , which would disturb his (her) normal sleep. When the patient defecates or coughs forcefully, the increased abdominal pressure is transmitted to the injured piriformis closely touching the sciatic nerve. Thus the pain would radiate down to the lower limb. The leg-straightened lifting test is positive below 60°; the pain is attenuated or disappears when the leg is lifted beyond 60°. The piriformis tension test (Fig. 170) is also positive. (The patient lies on his back, curving the knee and hip bone. The checker presses the knee with one hand and grasp the shank with the other to make the thigh adducted, making the piriformis in a tense state.).

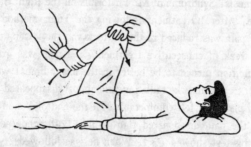

Fig. 170   Piriformis Tension Test

Tuina Manoeuvres

Principal methods: Manipulate by Rolling, Kneading with the Palm Base, Suppressing with the Flexed Elbow, Plucking, Pushing, and Straight-rubbing.

Subordinate methods: Apart from the tender spots, press and knead Huantiao (GB 30), Juliao (GB 29), Chengfu (BL 36), Yinmen (BL 37), Weizhong (BL 40), Chengshan (BL 57), and Yanglingquan (GB 34).

The treatment should be given once a day or every other day.

Case

Chang, male, 37, cadre. First visit: Feb. 20th, 1983.

Symptoms: Pain in the right arm, accompanied with radiating pain in the lower limbs for more than 3 months.

Case history: The patient got the morbid condition after by falling down from his bike. Being diagnosed as "prolapse of lumbar intrvertebral disc" and given such treatments as physiotherapy and traction, his condition did not take a turn for better; however, it got even worse, complicated by lame walking, malaise in the perineum, testicular atrophy and sexual impotence as well.

Physical examination: There was evident tenderness at the point Huantiao (GB 30) on the right side and muscular atrophy in the hip region; the piriformis test showed (+); sharp pain was felt when the leg-straightened lifting test showed 30° and disappeared when it showed 90°. No abnormal phenomenon was found on the X-ray examination.

Diagnosis: Syndrome of M. Piriformis on the Right Side.

Cure: After 1 treatment following the Tuina method mentioned above, pain was reduced in the buttock and the lower limb; after a whole week of consecutive treatment, the pain was greatly eased and condition turned to be better in the lower limbs; with another week of treatment, the radiating pain almost disappeared and the penis and perineum felt comfortable. At the end of 1 month of treatment, the pain disappeared thoroughly. Both tenderness and the piniformis test showed (−). When he was followed 2 years later, we got to know that he had recovered completely and resumed regular sexual behavior and work.

2. Injury of Superior Clunial Nerves

The superior nerves start from the lateral branch of the posterior ramus branch of spinal nerves of the 1st and 2nd lumbar vertebrae. They are distributed over the clunial surface through the lumbodorsal fascia (Fig. 171) and responsible for the sensation of the skin in that area.

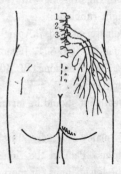

Etiology and Pathogenesis

Nerves below the iliac crese get injured easily when the body is frequently over-rotated, con-

Fig. 171 Superior Clunial Nerves

130

sequently resulting in deviation of the nerves from their original positions. Owing to that reason, aseptic inflammation, hyperemia, swelling and bleeding occur in the nerves and the tissues around.

Clinical Manifestations

There is evident pain in lumbar and hip regions unilaterally, especially in the area around the iliac crest. The pain may be dull, distending or stabbing and sometimes may radiated to the posterior thigh, aggravated when the patient bends his waist, turns the body or sits down. A subcutaneous nodular mass may be touchable in the soft tissue about 3－4 cm below the centre of the iliac crest, from which the patients suffer with pain, numbness and swelling. During the acute period, the orthotopia of the object may be found. The very tissue feel soft and thick, which reveals local tumerfaction. Similar object may also be felt in those chronically injured with slight tenderness, distension and numbness, however, most of the orthotopia has no clue to track.

Tuina Manoeuvres

Principal methods: Use Rolling, Kneading with the Palm Base, Revolving with the Forearm, Revolving with the Flexed Elbow, Suppressing with the Flexed Elbow and Pushing with the Palm.

Subordinate methods: Press and knead the nodular mass with both thumbs 1－2 times.

Case

Chang, male, 30, cadre. First visit: Apr. 20th, 1987.

Symptoms: Pain in the right portion of the waist and buttocks.

Case history: The patient got pain in his right lumbar gluteal region by sudden turning of the body during work a week ago. The pain and numbness radiated along the posterior side of the right thigh, getting more serious in case of squatting and standing as well as bending the waist. No effective result having been achieved with some casual treatment, things turned to be worse. Thus he came for help.

Physical examination: The lumbar vertebrae showed (－); a nodular mass was touchable 3 cm below the top of the iliac crest with evident tenderness.

131

Diagnosis: Trauma of the Right Superior Clunial Nerves

Cure: After 20 minutes of treatment, pain and numbness in the right lumbar gluteal region decreased immediately and bending the waist proved to be available. After 3 times of treatment, most symptoms mentioned above disappeared and the lumbar vertebra resumed its normal work, only with slight tenderness felt in the superior clinical nerves. Pain was completely removed from the diseased part of the body after 10 treatments and the tenderness vanished, which enabled the patient to resume his regular work. A year later we made following up and no recurrence was found.

3. Neuritis of Lateral Cutaneous Nerve of Thigh

The disease is also called meralgia. The lateral cutaneous nerve of the thigh, known as sensory nerve, starts from the posterior root of the spinal nerve of the 2nd, 3rd lumbar vertebrae. Protruding from the lateral greater psoas muscle, this nerve reaches the anterosuperior iliac spine across the deep surface of iliac muscle until it gets to the thigh by running below the inguinal ligament. Running below the lateral sartorias muscle, it pierces through the fascia at the point 5 — 10 cm away from the anterosuperior iliac spine and is divided into two branches, which reach the skin of the anterolateral thigh (Fig. 172).

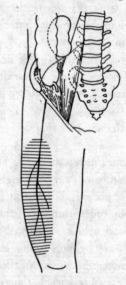

Fig. 172 Distribution of the Lateral Cutaneous Nerve of the Thigh

Etiology and Pathogenesis

In is believed that the disease is related to degeneration of the lumbar vertebrae; the fibrosis of local tissues tightens the nerve when it pierces through the fas-

132

cia lata, which also results in this disease. Some patients may get diseased by stimulation or oppression by reasons of tightening hard belt, carrying heavy objects in their pocket as well as pregnancy, hernia and visceraptosis, etc. In addition, attack of cold pathogens, infection, diabetes, excessive smoking, alcohol, poisoning and some vessel diseases such as arteriosc and varicosis of lower limbs may also cause neuritis of lateral cutaneous nerve of thigh.

Clinical Manifestations

The onset of the disease, which may be acute or chronic, usually takes place unilaterally. The symptoms may be paroxysm in those who are mildly diseased and turn to be persistent in those who are seriously diseased. The anterolateral skin perceives abnormal sensations as numbness, stiffness, burning and compression, accompanied with stabbing pain. Tender spots may be found within or below the anterosuperior iliac spine and different sizes and shapes of hypoesthetic area may appear on the anterolateral skin of the thigh.

Tuina Manoeuvres

Principal methods: Manipulate by Rolling, Kneading with the Palm Base, Grasping, Pressing, Knoching with the Fist and Straight-rubbing.

Subordinate methods: Press and knead Fengshi (GB 31), Biguan (ST 31), Futu (ST 32), Liangqiu (ST 34), and Yinlingquan (SP 9).

The operations should be carried out once day or once 2 days.

Case

Xu, female, 32. First visit: Feb. 15th, 1989.

Symptoms: Numb sensation on the anterolateral part of the right thigh for 2 months.

Case history: Slight tenderness was felt on the anterolateral side of the right thigh and within the right anterosuperior iliac spine. Sensation is reduced in the diseased part of the body yet the thigmesthesia remained normal.

Diagnosis: Neuritis of Lateral Cutaneous Nerve of the Right Thigh.

Cure: At the end of 1 Tuina treatment, such symptoms and signs as numbness and pain were relieved instantly; after 5 treatments, superficial sensibility resumed. With 13 treatments altogether, the patient was recovered. The patient was followed up for 4 years and no recurrence was found.

4. Sprain of Hip Joint

Etiology and Pathogenesis

The dominant factors for the disease are brutal over-extension or over-rotation of the hip region out of external force, i. e. , fall, stumble or jump with one foot landed. etc. Injuries of the hip region will bring about reactions of asceptic inflammation on the locale.

Clinical Manifestations

Owing to pain and swelling in the diseased area, the patient has to walk lamely with toes touching ground; furthermore, he (she) dare not straighten the affected hip joint when lying supine. There may find local tonic soft tissues and tenderness at the anterior medial aspect of the hip joint; and the pain may radiate from the medial aspect of the thigh to the knee, aggravated when the patient walks or flexes the hip joint with a force. The body temperature and erythrocyte sedimentation rate are both normal. On the X-ray examination, no abnormal phenomenon is found in the hip joint and its space. Tuina Manoeuvres

Principal methods: Adopt Rolling, Kneading with the Palm Base, Pressing, Plucking and Stretching in combination with passive movements of the hip joint.

Subordinate methods: In addition to the tender spots, press Biguan(ST 31), Futu (ST 32) and Fengshi (GB 31).

Stand by the affected side of the patient who is lying supine. First, dirigate with Rotating and Kneading with the Paine Base on the diseased part for several minutes; secondly, press the acupoints mentioned above until the arrival of Qi (the appearance of sore, numb, and distending sensation); thirdly, use Plucking to relieve spasm and convulsion of the tence muscles; finally perform Tuina therapy by counterextension (Fig. 173), lifting-up of the flexed lower limb(Fig. 174) and extorsion and abduction of the flexed hip joint until it extends (Fig, 175).

134

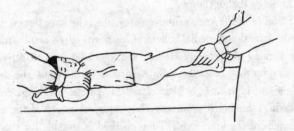

Fig. 173   Tuina Manoeuvre for Sprain of the
Hip Joint (1) Counterextension

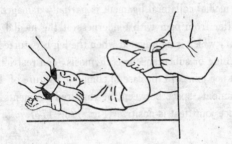

Fig. 174   Tuina Manoeuvre for Sprain of the
Hip Joint (2) Lifting-up Traction

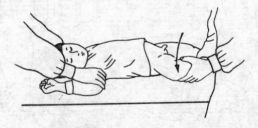

Fig. 175   Tuina Manoeuvre for Sprain of the
Hip Joint (3) Extorsion and Abduction

Perform the treatment once a day or once 2 days.

Trauma in Knees

1. Injury of Collateral Ligaments of Knee Joint

135

Etiology Pathogenesis

Stability of the knee joint decreases when the knee flexes. Injuries of the lateral and medial collateral ligaments often result from sudden turning of the body, falling and knocking in such activities as playing football or basketball. According to the traumatic degrees, 3 kinds of injuries have been classified: partial breaking, complete breaking, combined semilunar plate injury or injury of the cruciate ligament of the knee joint. Tuina method is suitable for those who have their ligaments sprained or partially lacerated.

Clinical Manifestations

When the medial collateral ligament is partially damaged, the patient will suffer from pain with tenderness at the medial aspect of the knee joint, which is aggravated when the leg is extorted passively, local swelling or subcutaneous ecchymosis, and restricted movement of the knee joint. In the case of complete rupture of the medial collateral ligament, space between the ruptured ligaments is touchable. The knee joint test is positive (Fig. 176—177).

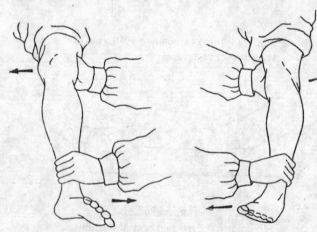

Fig. 176 Examination of the Medial Collateral Ligament of the Knee Joint

Fig. 177 Examination of the Lateral Collateral Ligament of the Knee Joint

Tuina Manoeuvres

Principal methods: Treat the disease by Round-rubbing, Kneading, Pressing, and Straight-rubbing.

Subordinate methods: Press and knead Dubi (ST 35), Xiyan (Ex —LE), Weizhong (BL 40), Liangqiu (ST 34), Xuehai (SP 10), Yinlingquan (SP 9), and Sanyinjiao (ST 6).

In the patient with evident pain, the strength applied should be mild and soft at first, and then increased with the subsidence of swelling and distension.

Perform the manoeuvres once a day or every 2 days.

Case

Yin, female, 47, cadre. First visit: Nov. 9th, 1990.

Case history: The patient got his left knee joint sprained 2 days ago, which resulted in pain at the medial aspect of the knee. She felt weak in the lower limbs and had difficulty in walking. As no effective result has been achieved with plaster, she came for Tuina manipulations.

Physical examination: It was found that the patient had low-graded swelling in the medial condyle of the left knee joint, evident tenderness, restricted activities of the knee joint, purplish tongue with whitish tongue coating, and tight wiry pulse. No abnormal phenomenon was shown on the X-ray examination.

Diagnosis: Injury of Lateral Collateral Ligament of the Left Knee Joint.

Cure: Pain was assuaged shortly after 20 minutes of Tuina treatment and the patient was able to walk freely. With 2 more treatments, the pain was got rid of thoroughly. Tenderness showed (−) and the knee joint could move flexibly. She recovered entirely half a month later.

2. Proliferative Gonitis

Proliferative gonitis is a chronic disease often encountered in old people, especially those who are obese. Delayed treatment may result in disturbance of the lower extremities.

Etiology and Pathogenesis

Senile tissue degeneration as well as frequent strain in the knee joint often leads to functional imbalance of the joint tension and the counter stress of the thigh bone, as well as decreased tolerance stress of the cartilage. Motivated by running, jumping and walking, the knee joint is prone to have spurs and osteopite resulting from protective new bone proliferation in the cartilage, joint capsule and ligament. It is shown in the statistic research that half of those who are over 40 years old have proliferation at various levels. Most people aged over 60 have spurs more or less and 20% of them have hyperemia, exudation and hydrops in their knee joint when chilled, sprained or overworked.

Clinical Manifestations

Pain occurs in the knee joint due to trauma or affection of cold. The pain often radiates to the knee-cap and the articular surface of the ossa cruris, and is aggravated in cold weather, damp residence, and overfatigue. The sound caused by friction can be heard when the knee joint moves. When the patient squats down, stands up or goes up and down, the cartilage may deviated from the articular cavity, causing the knee joint jammed and pain aggravated. X-ray examination reveals the formation of spurs, sharpening of the intercondyler eminence and stenosis of the space between the knee joint.

Tuina Manoeuvres

Principal methods: Rolling at the suprapatellar margin and quadriceps femoris (Fig. 178) for 3 minutes; knead the patella with the palm with increasing strength (Fig. 179); rub the medial aspect of the knee (Fig. 180); and roll the knee (Fig. 181) for 1—2 minutes. Afterwards adopt Nipping-grasping and Opening-shutting-rubbing for 0.5—1 minute respectively; and rolling at the popliteal fossa (Fig. 182) for 0.5—1 minute.

Subordinate methods: Press and knead Dubi (ST 35), Xiyan (Ex—LE), Xuehai (SP 10), Futu (ST 32), Fengshi (GB 31), Yanglingquan (GB 34), Yinlingquan (SP 9), Weizhong (BL 40) and Chengshan (BL 57).

Case

Liu, female, 62. First visit: May 7th, 1990.

Symptoms: Having pain in the left knee joint, she was limited in

138

squatting and standing up . Conditions turned to be worse 15 days ago.

Case history: Seven months prior to the onset of these symptoms, she felt soreness in the left knee joint, which was aggravated after long-distance walk and fatigue. Since her condition did not turn better with such treatments as oral pills, acupuncture therapy and physiotherapy, she came for Tuina manipulations.

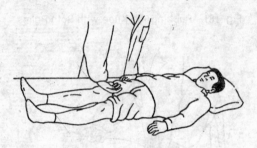

Fig. 178 Rolling at the Suprapatellar
Margin and Quadriceps Femoris

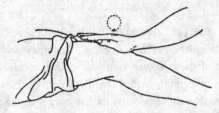

Fig. 179 Kneading the Patella with the Palm

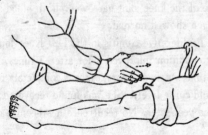

Fig. 180 Rubbing the Medial Aspect of the Knee

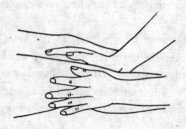

Fig. 181 Rubbing the Knee with Both Palms

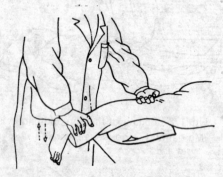

Fig. 182 Rolling at the Popliteal Fossa

Physical examination: Slight swelling, tenderness and disturbance of movement of the left knee joint were found in the examination. The X-ray examination revealed that hyperosteogeny existed at the tibia, and the lateral condyle and medial margin of the patella; the prominence between the condyles of the tibia became sharpened and the interspace of the knee joint narrowed. Both blood sedimentation and "O" antigen showed normal.

Diagnosis: Proliferative Gonitis in the Left Knee Joint.

Cure: Her condition improved a lot after 3 times of treatment. With 6 more times, pain and soreness was completely removed. The knee joint could curve freely. She was found recovered when we followed her up a year later. No recurrence has been heard ever since then.

3. Systremma

140

Etiology and Pathogenesis

Systremma may be caused by various factors, such as overfatigue of the lower limbs (a long-distance walk or riding of a bicycle),attack of cold (swimming in cold water without warming up), sudden strenuous exercises (running or jumping), or calciprivia during pregnancy.

Clinical Manifestations

The symptoms and signs of the disease are sudden convulsive pain in the calf of the affected leg with local prominence, difficulty in extending the lower limb, and disturbance of sleep by the convulsive sufferings.

Tuina Manoeuvres

Principal methods: Apply Grasping to the gastrocnemius muscle for 0.5 — 1 minute, then flex the ankle by pulling the toes (Fig. 183) for 1 — 2 minutes, and extend the ankle (Fig. 184) for 3 — 5 times.

Subordinate methods: Knead Weizhong (BL 40), and Chengshan (BL 57).

In most cases, pain can be relieved instantly by the manoeuvres mentioned-above.

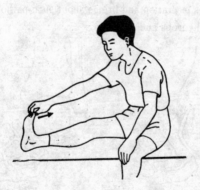

Fig. 183   Flexing the Ankle

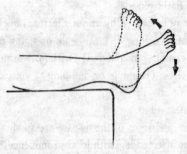

Fig. 184 Extending the Ankle

Injury of Ankle

1. Sprain of Ankle

Sprain of the ankle results from exertion of powerful tension on the lateral or medial ligaments out of sudden inward and outward turning of the ankle in walking, running or jumping. Those who are slightly injured have the ligament sprained or partly lacerated (Fig. 185) and those who are seriously diseased have their ligament completely lacerated (Fig. 186). In daily life inversion injury occurs most frequently, as the lateral malleolus is lower than the medial and the lateral ligament is thinner than the medial ligament, which usually causes laceration and brings about such pathological changes as bleeding, hydrops and adhesion.

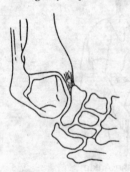

Fig. 185 Sprain of the Ligament of the Ankle Joint

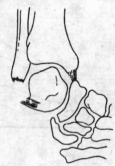

Fig. 186 Laceration of the Ligament of the Ankle Joint

142

Clinical Manifestations

Acute sprain is usually marked by evident swelling and pain in the ankle, tenderness at both lateral and medial aspects of the malleolus with a livid skin. For those who have their lateral mallelolus sprained, pain is aggravated when the ankle joint is turned inward. For those who injure their joint capsule, swelling occurs in the anterolateral or lower part of the malleolus. When the medial mellelolus is injured, fracture of the lateral mallelolus may also occur which brings about swelling and pain in both lateral and medial mallelolus. With fracture of lateral mallelotus, tenderness is found on the broken end where sharp pain is felt when the foot bottom is knocked, and friction sound is heard. Evident deform is also perceived in the ankle. Tuina method is suitable for those who have their soft tissues sprained in the ankle joint.

Tuina Manoeuvres

Principal methods: Use Round-rubbing, Kneading, Pressing, Pulling the Ankle, and Rotating the Ankle.

Subordinate methods: Press and knead Fengshi (GB 31), Zusanli (ST 36), Jiexi (ST 41), Taixi (KID 9), Kunlun (BL 60), Gongsun (SP 4), Xuanzhong (GB 39), and Taichong (LIV 3).

Ask the patient to lie on his (her) back. First, stroke and knead the diseased part and the shank for 2—3 minutes; then press and knead the acupoints mentioned-above for 0.5—1 minute respectively until the patient perceives the sensation of soreness, distention as well as numbness. After doing this, hold the patient's foot with the right hand and evert it to expand the medial space of the ankle joint; simultaneously press the space with the index finger of the left hand (Fig. 187) to expand its lateral space by enverting the ankle; afterwards swing the diseased foot slightly, inverting (Fig. 188) and extroverting (Fig. 189) for 1—2 times respectively.

For the patient with muscular spasm and articular adhesion, hold his (her) Achilles tendon with one hand and the foot with the other hand, and extend the ankle downwards (Fig. 190) before giving it sudden upward flexion (Fig. 191). Next, evert and invert the foot back (Fig. 192—193); rock the ankle for 3—5 times (Fig. 194) and rub it until the patient perceives a hot sensation.

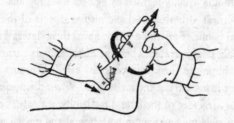

Fig. 187   Tuina Manoeuvre for Sprain of Ankle (1)

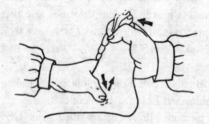

Fig. 188   Tuina Manoeuvre for Sprain of Ankle (2)

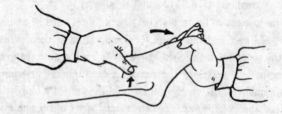

Fig. 189   Tuina Manoeuvre for Sprain of Ankle (3)

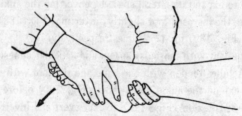

Fig. 190   Tuina Manoeuvre for Sprain of Ankle (4)

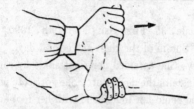

Fig. 191   Tuina Manoeuvre for Sprain of Ankle (5)

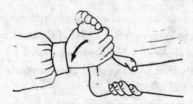

Fig. 192   Tuina Manoeuvre for Sprain of Ankle (6)

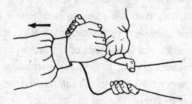

Fig. 193   Tuina Manoeuvre for Sprain of Ankle (7)

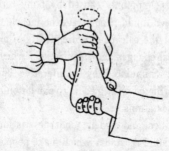

Fig. 194   Rotating the Ankle

145

Carry out the performance once a day or every other day.

Case

Chang, female, 35. First visit: Mar 19th, 1990.

Symptoms: Sprain of the right ankle for 1 day.

Case history: She sprained her right ankle by carelessness when she went downstairs the day before. She got acute pain in the lateral right ankle and could not touch land with her foot and neither could sleep well by suffering from sharp pain. She was accompanied to visit me.

Physical examination: Livid ecchymosis and swelling is perceived in the lateral and anterior inferior part of the right ankle respectively. Tenderness showed(+). Pain is aggravated when inversion occurs in the ankle joint. No abnormal phenomenon is found in the anteriorposterior and lateral film.

Diagnosis: Acute Sprain of the Right Ankle Joint.

Cure: Pain was relieved after 2 treatments according to the Tuina method mentioned-above and she could have a sound sleep at night. After 7 treatments, pain and swelling was mostly removed and the livid ecchymosis turned to be flavescent. Slight tenderness still existed in the anterior and lower part of the lateral mallelotus, yet the ankle joint resumed normal flexion and extension. With one more week of treatment, the ankle joint could move freely and the patient recovered a month later.

2. Calcaneal Spur

Etiology and Pathogenesis

The disease is commonly caused by bony retrograde affection, which is often seen in old people. As the muscle tendon attached to the tuberosity of the calcaneus is frequently stimulated, there will occur pathological changes and calcification, which may bring about hyperosteogeny. Stimulated by proliferative spurrs, the tissues around will be afflicted with bleeding, exudation and hydrops.

Clinical Manifestations

Pain is felt in heel and evident tenderness is found in medial heel as well as some solid reactant, which make people hardly stand and walk. Condition proves to be worse when people sit long, get out of

146

bed in the morning and walk, yet remitted after some movement and again, aggravated with fatigue. Certain old people does not have pain with their calcaneal spurs. The X-ray examination shows spurs have been formed at the end of the calcaneus as well as along its margins.

Tuina Manouevres

Principal methods: Apply Kneading the Tender Spot of the Heel with the Thumb (Fig. 195) for several minutes, Grasping to the gastrocnemius muscle, Knocking to the heel and Rotating the Ankle for 5—6 times respectively; finally, rub the affected part until the patient perceives a local burning sensation.

Subordinate methods: In addition to the tender spots, press and knead Jiexi (ST 41), Taixi (KID 9), Kunlun (BL 60), Sanyinjiao (ST 6), and Chengshan (BL 57).

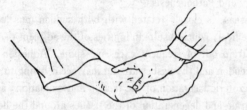

Fig. 195　Kneading the Tender Spot of the Heel

The treatment should be given once a day or every other day.

Case

Feng, female, 62. First visit: Sep. 25th, 1988.

Symptoms: Swelling pain in the right heel for a month.

Case history: Pain was felt in the right foot on Aug. 20th, 1988, which got serious 5 days later. The patient suffered from killing pain when she got out of bed in the morning and walked. Having been diagnosed as "Tuberosity of calcaneus bursities" in another hospital and given treatment with oral administration, she found her conditions remained the same. So she came to accept Tuina therapy.

Physical examination: Slight swelling was found in the right heel and the lower part of the medial mellelolus; tenderness was evident on and below the tuberosity of the calcaneus; motor function of the

147

right malleolus showed (−); the blood sendimendation was (−); the X-ray examination showed hyperosteogeny at the heel bottom as well as its margins .

Diagnosis: Right Calcaneal Spur.

Cure: Let the patient sit down. Press her tender spots for 3 minutes with the thumb, then knead the gastrocnemius muscle and knock the foot bottom for another 3 minutes, giving strength more and more. Shake 3−5 times the ankle joint and rub the foot bottom as well as the region around it until it gets hot. After 10 minutes of treatment, pain almost disappeared and only slight pain was felt when she landed forcefully. With 2 more weeks of therapy (1 treatment every two days), the patient could walk freely. No recurrence was found ever since.

3. Spain of Achilles Tendon

Etiology and Pathogenesis

This disease is closely related with both sudden muscle contraction in the heel, which results in injuries of the adjacent tissues, and gradual strain out of frequent excessive spots. Adhesion between Achilles tendon and the tissues around may occur owing to the acute sprain, acroteric laceration of the tendon and exudation, as well as chronic strain and degeneration of the tissues around the heel.

Clinical Manifestations

The disease is chiefly marked by achillodynia, which, however, relieved with some movement and aggravated when people jump or run forcefully. As it becomes more and more serious, pain is felt whenever Achilles tendon is moved (going upstairs or downstairs, etc.)and sharpens when Achilles tendon is pressed. Deformity of Achilles tendon may occur in the later stage and a gelosis, named " tenosynovitis", is touchable on the surface, which results in loss of tenacity and elasticity of the tendon.

Tuina Manouevres

Principal methods: Adopt the following manouevres on the diseased lower limb: Rolling, Kneading, Twisting, Grasping, Rotating the Ankle, Flexing the Ankle and Extending the Ankle (Fig. 184), focused on the Achilles tendon and shank of the diseased side.

Subordinate methods: Apart from the tender spots, press and knead Kunlun (BL 60), Jiexi (ST 41), Taixi (KID 9), Xuanzhong (GB 39), Chengshan (B 57), Sanyinjiao (ST 6), and Gongsun (SP 4).

Internal Medicine

1. Common Cold

Common cold, also called "catching cold", means inflammation of the upper respiratory tract, which often occurs in winter and spring.

Etiology and Pathogenesis

This disease results mainly from attack of the Lung by Pathogenic Wind. It is often classified into two types: Wind-Cold and Wind-Heat. Clinical Manifestations

Common cold due to Wind-Cold: Marked by aversion to cold, fever, headache, pyrexia without perspiration, soreness and pain of the limbs, stuffy nose, watery nasal discharge, white and thin coating of the tongue, and floating tight pulse.

Common cold due to Wind-Heat: Marked by severe pyrexia with little perspiration, slight aversion to cold, dry mouth, sore-throat, general heaviness sensation, red tip of the tongue with thin and yellowish coating, and floating rapid pulse.

Tuina Manoeuvres

Principal methods: Push and rub the neck, shoulder and back (see Fig. 196); knead and grasp the neck (Fig. 197); afterwards, push Yintang (Ex－HN) (Fig. 198), push the superciliary arch (Fig. 199) with the two thumbs, and knead Taiyang (Ex－HN) (Fig. 200) 30－50 times respectively.

In addition to the above-mentioned manipulations, when the case pertains to Wind-Cold type, Opening-shutting-rubbing, Scraping, and Scratching are needed; when it belongs to Wind-Heat type,

Tapping is necessary; when the patient is afflicted with general aching, Grasping of the four limbs should be applicable.

Subordinate methods: Press and knead Fengchi (GB 20), Fengfu (DU 16), Fengmen (BL 12), Jianjing (GB 21), Quchi (LI 11), and Hegu (LI 14). In the case with headache, plus Baihui (DU 20); in the case with watery nasal discharge, plus Yingxiang (LI 20).

Carry out the dirigation once a day or every other day.

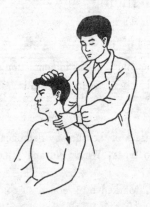
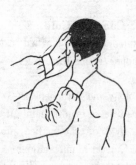

Fig. 196   Pushing-rubbing
the Neck, Shoulder and
Back

Fig. 197   Kneading-grasping
the Neck

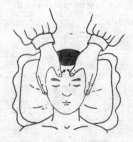

Fig. 198   Pushing Yintang
(Ex-HN) with Both Thumbs

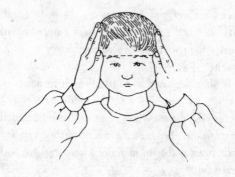

Fig. 199 Pushing the Superciliary
Arch with Both Thumbs

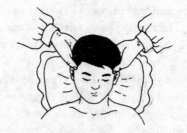

Fig. 200 Kneading Taiyang (Ex-HN)

Case

Qi, male, 37. First visit: May 7th, 1988.

Symptoms: Aversion to cold, watery nasal discharge and soreness of the head and aching of the whole body.

Case history: The patient caught cold 2 days ago during night sleep and he got pain in the head and the whole body, stuffy running watery nose as well as rigidity and malaise of the cervical and back regions. No effective result having been achieved with oral administration of APC, he came for Tuina treatment.

Physical examination: Low and hoarse voice, temperature at 37. 2 C with no perspiration, slight tenderness of the muscles in the back and four limbs, thin and white coating of the tongue, floating and tight pulse.

Diagnosis: Common Cold due to Wind-Cold.

151

Cure: After 20 minutes of 1 treatment, the body sweated a little and the stuffy nose and aching all over was reduced. With another day's treatment, the patient recovered completely.

2. Headache

Headache is often seen in clinical practice. It responds well to Tuina therapy when it is not caused by the following factors: intracranial space-occupying disease, contusion or laceration of the brain, traumatic intracranial hemotoma, pyencephalus cerebrovascular, etc. Tuina is more suitable to migraine, headache due to myophagism or hypertension.

Etiology and Pathogenesis

Traditionally, the disease is divided into two subcategories: headache due to exogenous pathogenic factors, and headache due to internal injury. The first is closely related to Pathogenic Wind and Cold, Wind and Heat, Summer Dampness, which result in Qi and Blood Stagnation. The second results mainly from Kidney Deficiency and Blood Deficiency as well as Liver Yang Rising, which lead to loss of nutrients in the brain. In addition, headache may be brought about by Turbid Phlegm, which fails to prevent Lucid Yang from rising and Turbid Yin from descending; it may also be caused by trauma, which leads to Blood Stasis, consequently obstruction in the mental Collaterals so that Qi and Blood can not flow freely.

Clinical Manifestations

Headache due to Wind-Cold: Manifested by pain in the head, which radiates to the neck and back, often accompanied with aversion to cold, preference for covering the head, no perspiration, thin and whitish tongue coating, and floating and tight pulse.

Headache due to Wind-Heat: Marked by distending pain in the head, fever, aversion to cold, thirst, sore-throat, dark urine, red tongue tip, yellowish thin coating of the tongue and floating rapid pulse.

Headache due to Summer Dampness: Marked by tight pain in the head, oppressed feeling in the chest, lassitude of the limbs, pyrexia with perspiration , vexation, thirst, white and greasy fur and soft moderate pulse.

Headache due to Kidney Deficiency: Characterized by hollow pain in the head, dizziness, tinnitus, soreness and weakness of the loins and lower limbs, impotence, thin and white fur, pale tongue, and deep thread pulse.

Headache due to Blood Deficiency: Marked by dizziness, sallow and dim complexion, lassitude, listlessness, palpitation and shortness of breath, pale tongue, thin and yellow tongue as well as thread and weak pulse.

Headache due to Liver Yang Rising: Shown as distending pain in the head, vertigo, giddiness, vexation, irritability, insomnia, distending pain in chest region, redness of tongue with thin and yellow coating, and wiry thread pulse.

Headache due to Turbid Phlegm: Marked mainly by pain in the head, fullness and distention in the chest and hypotrondrium, excessive expectoration, white and greasy coating of the tongue, and slippery pulse.

Headache due to Blood Stasis: Characterized with fixed pricking pain in the head, purplish dark tongue with ecchymosis sometimes, and uneven pulse.

Tuina Manoeuvres

Principal methods: Use Pushing the Forehead Divergently, Wiping, Pinching the Eyebrows, Kneading with the Finger, Grasping with the Five Fingers, Pushing-wiping and Rotating.

Subordinate methods: Press and knead the tender spots, Yintang (Ex—HN), Taiyang (Ex—HN), Yuyao (Ex—HN), Touwei (ST 8), Baihui (DU 20), Fengfu (DU 16), Fengchi (GB 20), Quchi (LI 11), Hegu (LI 14), Hegu (LI 14), Lieque (LI 7), and Zusanli (ST 36).

Apart from the above routine manipulations, knead Feishu (BL 13), Fengmen (BL 12), and Jianjing (GB 21) in the case of Wind-Cold; press Dazhui (DU 14) in Wind-Heat type; grasp Jianjing (GB 21), and Hegu (LI 14) in the case of Summer Dampness; knead Shenshu (BL 23) and Mingmen (DU 4) in Kidney Deficiency; press and knead Zhongwan (REN 12), Qihai (REN 6) and Guanyuan (REN 4) in Blood Deficiency; push Qiaogong (Bridge Arch, along sternocleidomastoid muscle at both sides of the neck) (Fig. 201) from above on either side of the neck for 20 times, then press Taichong (Liv 3), in the case of Liver Yang Rising; knead Pishu (BL 20), Weishu (BL 21), and Dachangshu (BL 25) in the case of Turbid Phlegm; rub the forehead, and press either Taiyang (Ex — HN) in the case of Blood Stasis.

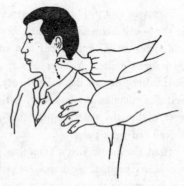

Fig. 201   Pushing Qiaogong (the Bridge Arch)

The manipulations should be carried out once a day or every other day.

Case

Liu, male, 53. First visit: Mar. 8th, 1993.

Symptoms: Distending pain in the head, accompanied with vertigo for 7 days.

Case history: The patient had severe headache in the forehead and left portion of the head, combined with dizziness, feeling of fullness in the head, soreness and pain in the nape and back region, insomnia and dreaming. Having been treated with piminodine, the patient still suffered a lot. Thus she came for Tuina therapy.

Physical examination: There occurred tenderness in either Taiyang (Ex — HN). The rheoencephalogram revealed a verte-brobasilar pulsating ischenica. The X-ray examination showed slight hyperosteogeny in the 5th, 6th and 7th anterior magin. The tongue was red with thin yellow fur. The pulse was tight.

Diagnosis: Headache due to Liver Yang Rising.

Cure: After 15 minutes of 1 treatment, the pain was instantly relieved. With 3 more treatments, all his symptoms disappeared.

3. Insomnia

Etiology and Pathogenesis

The disease results from the following factors: impairment of the

154

Heart and Spleen and exhaustion of Heart Blood by long-term depression, which leads to Deficiency of the Heart and Spleen; chronic illness, excessive sexual life, which result in consumption of Kidney Yin and incoordination of the Heart and Kidney, thus Deficiency of Fire; improper diet and indigestion which damage the Intestines and Stomach, thus producing Phlegm Heat; irritation and annoyance which impairs the Liver, thus leading to the Stagnation of Liver Qi.

Clinical Manifestation

Insomnia due to Heart-Spleen Deficiency: Marked by disturbance of sleep at night, excessive dream, amnesia, palpitation, lassitude, listlessness, anorexia, dim complexion, pale tongue, thin and whitish fur, thread and weak pulse.

Insomnia due to Deficiency of Fire: Manifested by d'sturbance of sleep at night, vexation, dizziness, tinnitus, Heat sensation in palms and soles, dry mouth and dry tongue, palpitation, amnesia, soreness of the loins, nocturnal emission, red tongue with little coating as well as a thread and rapid pulse.

Insomnia due to Phlegm Heat: Marked by disturbance of sleep at night, oppressed feeling in the chest, heaviness in the head, fidgets, bitter taste, dizziness, yellowish greasy tongue coating, and slippery rapid pulse.

Insomnia due to Liver Qi Stagnation: Characterized by disturbance of sleep at night, constipation, red tongue with yellow coating and tight rapid pulse.

Tuina Manoeuvres

Principal methods: Treat the disease by Wiping, Pressing, Kneading, Grasping Pushing the Forehead Divergently, Pinching the Eyebrows, Pushing-wiping and Pinching along the Spine.

Subordinate methods: Press and knead Yintang (Ex—HN), Jingming (BL 1), Zanzhu (BL 2), Taiyang (Ex—HN), Fengchi (GB 20), Jianjing (GB 21), Zhongwan (REN 12), Qihai (REN 6) and Guanyuan (REN 4).

In addition, in the case of Heart-Spleen Deficiency, rub the left portion of the back horizontally (Fig. 202), and knead Xinshu (BL 15), Pishu (BL 20), Weishu (BL 21) and Zusanli (ST 36); in the case of Deficiency of Fire, knead Shenshu (BL 23), Mingmen (DU 4), Yongquan (KID 1) (Fig. 203) and push Qiaogong (Bridge Arch); in the case of Phlegm Heat, knead Fenglong (ST 40), Pishu (BL 20) and Weishu (BL 21).

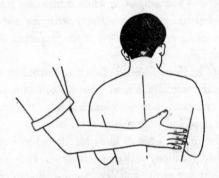

Fig. 202   Rubbing the Left Portion
of the Back Horizontally

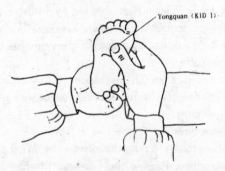

Yongquan (KID 1)

Fig. 203   Kneading Yongquan (KID 1)

Perform the Tuina therapy once a day or every other day.

Case

Yang, female, 40. First visit: Sep. 25th, 1989.

Symptoms: Suffering from insomnia for 2 years, which was aggravated for half a year.

Case history: The patient got diseased 2 years ago by excessive anxiety with symptoms such as excessive dreaming during sleep, anorexia, general debility, palpitation and amnesia. Having been diagnosed as neurosism and given treatment of oral acanthapanaxroot and diazepam, the disease remained the same. For the last 6 months, her condition got worse and she could only enjoy 3 – 4 hours of sleep each day.

Physical examination: A middle-aged woman with sallow and dim complexion; pathologic leanness; abdominal distention; pink tongue with thin and white coating; thread and feeble pulse. The barium meal fluoroscopy report diagnosed it as chronic gastritis.

Diagnosis: Insomnia due to Heart-Spleen Deficiency.

Cure: After 30 minutes of 1 treatment, the patient got 5 – 6 hours of sleep at the very night; after 3 treatments, she got 7 hours of sleep and did not dream at night; after 12 treatments she got normal sleep and recovered completely a month later.

4. Hiccup

Hiccup refers to upward adverse flow of Qi causing short and frequent sound which can not be easily controlled.

Etiology and Pathogenesis

The dominant factors for the disease are excess of cold raw food or Cold-producing drugs, which bring about retention of Cold in the Stomach and failure of descending Stomach Qi; stimulation by depressed emotions, which arrives at transverse attack of diaphragm by the upward adverse flow of Liver Qi; serious or protracted illness which leads to Vital Qi Deficiency and Stomach Qi Insufficiency.

Clinical Manifestations

Hiccup due to Stomach Cold is marked by slow and powerful hiccup sound, malaise in the upper abdomen, which is relieved with warmth and aggravated with cold, no thirst, anorexia, thin and whitish tongue coating, and slow moderate pulse.

Hiccup due to Liver Qi Rising is characterized by continuous hiccups which is beyond self-control and is aggravated when in anxiety or indignation, accompanied by fidgets, oppressed feeling in the chest, white thin coating of the tongue, and wiry pulse.

Hiccup due to Vital Qi Deficiency is marked by low and weak hiccup sound, shortness of breath, pale complexion, cold limbs, lassitude, anorexia, pale tongue with thin and white coating, and thready, deep and weak pulse.

Tuina Manoeuvres

Principal methods: Use Pressing, Kneading and Straight-rubbing.

Subordinate methods: Press and knead Geshu (BL 17), Shanzhong (REN 17), Zhongwan (REN 12), Neiguan (PC 6), and Taichong (LIV 3).

In addition to the manoeuvres mentionedabove, rub the left portion of the back horizontally until there appears a local warm sensation, then press Pishu (BL 20) and Weishu (BL 21), in the case of Stomach Cold; knead Zhangmen (LIV 13) and Qimen (LIV 14) in the case of Liver Qi Rising; press and knead Zusanli (ST 36) and pinch the spine in the case of Vital Qi Deficiency.

Case

Chang, female. 32. First visit: Apr. 15th, 1989.

Symptoms: Continuous hiccup for 2 days.

Case history: She got hiccups by emotional stimulation 2 days earlier, which could not be controlled and accompanied with short and continues sound. Meanwhile she got irritability and eructation. Oral administration of the traditional Chinese medicine failed to improve her condition. So she came for Tuina treatment.

Physical examination: Hiccup with loud sound; fidgets and restlessness; thin and yellowish tongue coating and tight pulse.

Diagnosis: Hiccup due to Liver Qi Rising.

Cure: After 5 minutes of 1 treatment, the hiccup stopped instantly and the patient resumed normal work. She was followed up a week later and was found recovered completely. No recurrence was heard.

5. Epigastralgia

Epigastralgia is a disease of the digestive canal tract marked by pain in the upper part of the abdomen. Also called "cardiac ache", it often occurs along with such diseases as gastritis, gastrelcoma and gastrospasm, etc.

Etiology and Pathogenesis

158

The main factors for the disease are as follows: affection of the Stomach by accumulation of exopathic cold or excess of cold raw food, leading to retention of Cold in the Stomach; excessive heat-producing food (greasy or sweet food), leading to impairment of the Stomach; stimulation of emotions, leading to Liver Qi Stagnation and then adverse upward flow of Liver Qi, which attacks the Stomach; overfatigue or improper diet, leading to Insufficiency of the Spleen and Stomach, thus weakened function of the Stomach in receiving and digesting food.

Clinical Manifestations

Epigastralgia due to Stomach Cold: Marked mainly by a sudden pain in the epigastric region, preference for warmth and hot drinks, no thirst, watery vomitus, loss of appetite, loose stool, whitish thin tongue coating as well as wiry tight pulse.

Epigastralgia due to Stomach Heat: Marked by distending pain in the upper abdomen, polydipsia, halitosis, belching, acid regurgitation, retention of the undigestive food with alleviation after vomiting, constipation, as well as greasy tongue coating and slippery pulse.

Epigastralgia due to Liver Qi Rising: Characterized with distention and pain in the upper abdomen, radiating to the hypochondriac regions, belching, fidgets, restlessness, and wiry pulse.

Epigastralgia due to Insufficiency of the Spleen and Stomach: Manifested by dull pain and fullness in the Stomach, anorexia, dyspepsia, preference for warmth and pressure, cold limbs, and loose bowels, and pale lips and tongue.

Tuina Manoeuvres

Principal methods: Perform the following on the abdomen: On-the-point-pressing, Pressing, Kneading with the Thenar Eminence, Round-rubbing and Grasping; manipulate by Pressing and Kneading from Dazhui(DU 14) to Sanjiaoshu (BL 22) along the course of the Bladder Channel on the back; use Pressing, Kneading and Grasping on the back, shoulders and upper limbs.

Subordinate methods: Press and knead Zhongwan (REN 12), Qihai (REN 6), Tianshu (ST 25), Zusanli (ST 36), Ganshu (BL

18), Pishu (BL 20), Weishu (BL 21), Jianjing (GB 21), Shousanli (LI 10), Neiguan (PC 6), and Hegu (LI 14).

Moreover, knead the left portion of the back in the case of Stomach Cold; stroke his (her) abdomen clockwise in Stomach Heat; rub and stroke the hypotrondriac regions (Fig. 204), knead Zhangmen (LIV 13) and Qimen (LIV 14) in the case of Liver Qi Rising.

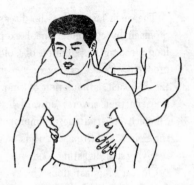

Fig. 204 Rubbing the Hypotrondria

Carry out the manoeuvres once a day or every other day.

Case

Sun, female, 38. First visit: Feb. 20th, 1985.

Symptoms: Frequent pain attack to the upper abdomen for more than 2 years, aggravated for 15 days.

Case history: Stimulated emotionally 2 years ago, the patient got excessive anxiety and irregular diet, which caused distention and pain in the Stomach radiating to the hypochondric region. She suffered a lot after meal with the symptoms such as belching, nausea, etc. No satisfactory effect having been achieved with oral administration of probanthine, she came for Tuina therapy.

Physical examination: Tenderness (+) in the upper abdomen; slight distention of the Stomach; red tongue with thin whitish coating and wiry pulse.

Diagnosis: Epigastralgia due to Liver Qi Rising.

Cure: Having been pressed at the tender spot for 2 minutes, the patient got the pain greatly relieved; after 6 treatments, the pain almost disappeared. With 2 more weeks of Tuina treatment, she recovered thoroughly. No recurrence was found in the following 2 years.

6. Gastroptosia

Gastroptosia is a chronic disease which occurs when the lowest arc

160

line of the Stomach lesser curvature drops below iliac crest line or duodenal bulb and deviates to the left.

Etiology and Pathogenesis

The disease is presupposed by the following factors: improper diet as well as excessive activities after meal, leading to damage of the Spleen and Stomach; impairment of Seven Emotions, resulting Liver Qi Stagnation, the transverse attack of Liver Qi, consumption of Vital Qi, sinking of Spleen Qi, which fails to elevate the Stomach. Such factors as delivery, prolonged illness may also lead to Qi and Blood Deficiency, consumption of Vital Qi and weakened function of the Stomach and Spleen, thus the disease.

Clinical Manifestations

Most patients get lean figure, with the lower abdomen protruding. Abdominal pain is often felt and distending sensation appears after meal. Sometimes, the patient has constipate, diarrhoea and loose bowels, in combination with dizziness, debility, palpitation, insomnia, etc. Strong pulsation may be felt at the upper abdomen. The barium meal fluoroscopy shows the Stomach drops when the patient stands up and the tensile force decreases.

Tuina Manoeuvres

Principal methods: Apply Round-rubbing, Pressing, and Vibrating to the abdomen; use Rolling (along the course of the Bladder Channel), Pressing, Kneading and Inserting on the back.

Subordinate methods: Press and knead Zhongwan (REN 12), Qihai (REN 6), Tianshu (ST 25), Pishu (BL 20), Weishu (BL 21) and Ganshu (BL 18).

In the patients with Qi and Blood Deficiency, rub the Du Channel on the left portion of the back horizontally until the patient perceives a burning sensation on the affected locale, then pinch the spine and knead Zusanli (ST 36); in the patients with Liver Qi Stagnation, knead Zhangmen (LIV 13), Qimen (LIV 14) and Taichong (LIV 3) as well.

Perform the manipulations once a day or every other day.

7. Arthralgia

Arthralgia refers to such symptoms as pain, soreness, heaviness and numbness occurring in muscles, tendons and joints, as well as arthrocele and rigidity of joints, etc.

Etiology and Pathogenesis

The disease results mostly from general asthenia, imbalance of Ying and Wei Levels, attack of Wind-Cold-Dampness; or hyperactivity of Yang and retention of Heat in the body; or Deficiency of Fire, which produces Yang Rising when meeting with Pathogenic Cold, thus leading to the affection of the Channels and Collaterals in the joint.

Clinical Manifestations

Arthralgia due to Wind-Cold-Dampness: When pathological changes occur in the joint, there will be pain, soreness and numbness in the joint, aggravated with weather changes, thin and whitish tongue coating, wiry tight or soft moderate pulse. When they occur in muscles, the symptoms are general pain, numbness of the muscles, thickening of sweat pores, whitish and greasy tongue coating, soft and moderate pulse. When affected mainly by Pathogenic Wind, the patient is prone to suffer from wandering pain; when affected mainly by Pathogenic Cold, he is prone to get fixed pain with numbness of the extremities.

Arthralgia due to Heat: The morbid state is marked by pain of joints, circumscribed redness, swelling and burning sensation, assuaged by cold, difficulty in joint movement, wandering pain which may involve one joint or more, complicated by fever with sweating, aversion to wind, dire thirst, reddened tongue with yellowish or dry coating and slippery rapid pulse.

Tuina Manoeuvres

Principal methods: Use the following manoeuvres around the affected area: Rolling, Kneading, Grasping, Round-rubbing, Twisting, Rotating, Rubbing with Both Palms and Shaking.

Subordinate methods: Press and knead Jianjing (GB 21), Quchi (LI 11), Hegu (LI 14); Feishu (BL 13), Shenshu (BL 23), and Dachangshu (BL 25); Huantiao (GB 30), Yanglingquan (GB 34), Yinlingquan (SP 9) and Kunlun (BL 60); Baihui (DU 20), Fengchi (GB 20) and Fengfu (DU 16).

162

Carry the performance out once a day or every other day.

Case

Liu, male, 43. First visit: Dec. 29, 1987.

Symptoms: Pain in the shoulder and back regions for more than one year, aggravated for 3 months.

Case history: Being chilled 1 year ago, the patient got heavy, sore pain in his right shoulder and back region, aggravated with cold and relieved with heat. Having been treated with oral administration as bruffen, indomethacim and chaenomeles fruit, he did not feel better, thus he came for help.

Physical examination: Movement is possible in the neck, shoulder and elbow; tenderness shows (+) at Tianzong (SI 11). Analysis report: mucin 45 mg; normal blood sedimentation; normal result on the X-ray examination of the cervical vertebrae. The tongue got thin and whitish fur; the pulse was thread.

Diagnosis: Arthralgia due to Wind-Cold-Dampness.

Cure: After 20 minutes of 1 treatment, pain in the right body was instantly relieved and almost disappeared after 3 treatments. The neck, shoulder and elbow resumed flexible movement. After 3 more treatments, all symptoms disappeared. He was found recovered when he was followed up half a year later and no recurrence had been heard.

8. Hypertension

Hypertension is a common chronic disease marked by continual increase of arterial pressure. Generally speaking, when people are in rest, blood pressure over 18. 7/12 kPa or diastolic pressure over 13. 3 kPa may be viewed as hypertension.

Etiology and Pathogenesis

This disease is closely associated with such factors as long-term mental stress and irritability, which bring about Liver Qi Stagnation and Fire Deficiency which lead to Liver Yang Rising. It is also associated with Kidney Yin Insufficiency for overfatigue or old age. In addition, irregular diet or too greasy food as well as drinking too much, which may cause Turbid Phlegm and thus the obstruction of the Channels and Collaterals, may also result in the disease.

Clinical Manifestations

Hypertension is usually classified as two types: the benign and the malignant. Clinically, the former occurs more frequently.

Benign hypertension: The morbid state is usually manifested by headache, dizziness, insomnia, hypoprosexia, hypomnesis, fidgets, asthenia, palpitation, etc. There may occur pathological changes in the Heart, brain and Kidney at the later stage.

Malignant hypertension: It is marked by an acute onset from the benign type, or accidental occurrence, often seen in people under 40 years old. The blood pressure increases rapidly, with the diastolic pressure above 17.3 — 18.7 kPa. In months or 1 — 2 years, pathological changes would occur in the Kidney or Heart. Patients of this type of hypertension are easily afflicted with encephalopathy, Heart failure and sudden decrease of renal functions.

Tuina Manoeuvres

Principal methods: Push Qiaogong (the Bridge Arch) (Fig. 205) from above, first on the left side then on the right for 20 — 30 times respectively; then use Wiping, Pushing the Forehead Divergently, Pushing-wiping, Grasping with the Five Fingers, Kneading-grasping the Upper Limbs (Fig. 206), Kneading with the Finger, Pushing the Back with both Palms (Fig. 207), Kneading-grasping the Posterior Aspect of the Lower limbs (Fig. 208), Straight-rubbing on the lumbosacral portion and at Yongquan (KID 1).

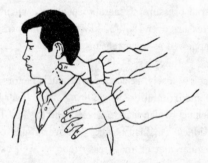

Fig. 205 Pushing Qiaogong (the Bridge Arch)

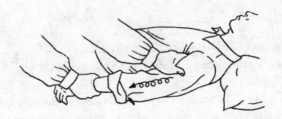

Fig. 206 Kneading-grasping the Upper Limbs

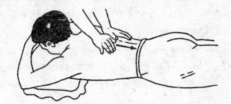

Fig. 207 Pushing the Back with Both Palms

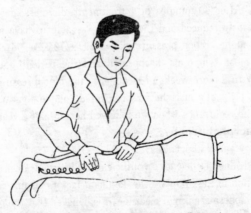

Fig. 208 Kneading-grasping the Posterior
Aspect of the Lower Limbs

Subordinate methods: Press and knead Yintang (Ex − HN),
Taiyang (Ex − HN), Baihui (DU 20), Fengchi (GB 20), Fengfu
(DU 16), Touwei (ST 8), Gongsun (SP 4), Zanzhu (BL 2),
Dazhui (DU 14), Guanyuan (REN 4), Qihai (REN 6), Zhongwan
(REN 12), Shenshu (BL 23), Mingmen (DU 4), Yongquan (KID

165

1).

Case

Qu, female, 53. First visit: May 19th, 1982.

Symptoms: Headache, dizziness, and heaviness in the head for 3 years.

Case history: The patient was afflicted with the following symptoms and signs for three years: dizziness, migraine, heaviness distension of the head, insomnia, dreaminess as well as hypomnesis. Having been diagnosed as "neurosism" and treated with oral administration of traditional Chinese medicine, she still suffered a lot. So she came for Tuina therapy.

Physical examination: It was found that the patient got blood pressure 21. 9/13. 3 kPa, red tongue with thin yellowish fur, thread pulse. Besides, left ventricular hypertrophy is visible through the electrocardiogram.

Diagnosis: Hypertension due to Liver Yang Rising.

Cure: After 30 minutes of 1 treatment, dizziness and headache was instantly reduced and the patient was able to have a six-hour sleep at night. Blood pressure shows 19. 9/12 kPa; after 4 treatments, most symptoms disappeared and the patient got a sound sleep. With 2 more weeks of treatment, the bloodpressure lowered to 18. 6/11. 9 kPa and she was recovered completely. We learned she had no recurrence when we followed her up half a year later.

9. Encephalatrophy

Etiology and Pathogenesis

Senile Kidney Deficiency, insufficiency of reservoir of marrow and malnutrition in the brain are the dominant factors leading to the disease. In modern science of medicine, it is believed that the pathological changes of the disease are as follows: diffuse atrophy of the brain tissues, stenosis of convolution, deep and broad cerebral grooves.

Clinical Manifestations

The disease is often manifested as dizziness, staggering walking, clumsiness in movement, hypomnesis and decrease in working ability. With the progression of the disease, there may occur loss of memory, asophia and apathy, unclear enunciation, apathetic expression, at last inability to get up and dementia. It is found by examination that the patient keeps stumbling and has his hypermyotonia raised. Rromberg's sign, the finger-nose test, quick diadochokinetic test and heel-knee-tibia test are all positive. The syndrome of encephalatrophy is visible through CT scanning of the cerebral cranium.

Tuina Manoeuvres

Principal methods: Treat the disease by Pushing the Forehead Divergently, Wiping, Pinching the Eyebrows, Grasping with the Five Fingers, Pushing-wiping, Stroking-grasping (Benefiting the Brain), Kneading with the Finger and Opening-shutting-rubbing.

Subordinate methods: Press and knead Zanzhu (BL 2), Taiyang (Ex−HN), Jingming (BL 1), Yintang (Ex−HN), Sibai (ST 2), Shangxing (DU 23), Baihui (DU 20), Lieque (LI 7), Zusanli (ST 36), Shenshu (BL 23)and Mingmen (DU 4).

The treatment should be given once a day or every other day.

Case

Wang, male, 59, cadre. First visit: Aug. 20th, 1991.

Symptoms: Dizziness, hypomnesis and habitude for 3 months or so.

Case history: The patient got the symptoms and signs mentioned-above 3 months ago. Being diagnosed as dementia and treated with vitamin E and pyrithioxine, the disease did not take a turn for the better at all, and recently it became more serious. So he came for help.

Physical examination: Blood pressure 16/10 kPa, normal activity of the Heart and Lung, regular diet, pink tongue with thin and white fur, deep, thread and weak pulse.

Diagnosis: Encephalatrophy.

Cure: After 1 treatment for 20 minutes, his mind was tranquilized and dizziness evidently relieved. After 2 weeks of Tuina dirigation, he could walk steadily and got a better memory. With 1 more month of treatment, the symptoms almost disappeared and he resumed normal work. He was found thoroughly recovered when followed up half a year later.

10. Hemiplegia

Hemiplegia refers to such symptoms and signs as paralysis in limbs and face unilaterally, stiff tongue, etc. In most cases, it is a sequel of apoplexy; it may also be caused by encephalatrophy or trauma.

Etiology and Pathogenesis

According to the Chinese medicine, hemiplegia is closely related to Deficiency of Fire, and Phlegm-Dampness in the body, which lead to Liver Yang Rising and up-stirring of Liver Wind.

Clinical Manifestations

The disease is commonly manifested by unilateral paralysis of the limbs, deviation of the mouth and eye, tongue rigidity, retardation in speech. At its initial stage, the patient suffers from weakness of the limbs, dysesthesia, disturbance of limb movement; later there will occur severe rigidity, contracture and deformity in the affected limb. Hypermyotonia, decrease of superficial sensibility and muscular atrophy can be found through examination.

Hoffmann's sign: Hold the wrist of the patient and slightly curve the fingers. Grip the patient's middle finger with the index and middle fingers of the right hand, then pluck and scrape the nail of the patient downwards with the thumb nail rapidly (Fig. 209). With an inward flexion of the thumb and other three fingers, the patient is proved to have positive reaction.

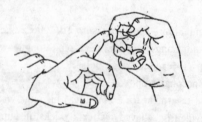

Fig. 209 Hoffmann's sign

Ankle-clonus test: Arrange the patient to lie on his back with his hip joint and knee joint flexed. Support the patient's popliteal fossa

168

with one hand, fix the farther end of the foot with the other hand, then flex and extend the ankle joint powerfully with high frequency (Fig. 210). Rhythmical movements of the ankle joint means positive reaction.

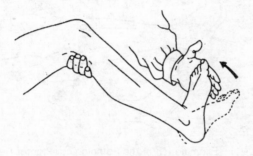

Fig. 210   Ankle-clonus Test

Babinski's sign: Starting from the heel, draw lines at the foot bottom with a bamboo spike along the lateral side to the medial side via the little toe. Everything goes normal if the toes flex toward'the foot bottom (Fig. 211 (1)). But if the big toe flexes towards its dorsum and the others extend dispersinly, the test shows positive (Fig. 211(2)).

Oppenheim sign: Rub the anterior shank with the belly of a thumb along the anterior side of the tibia (Fig. 211 (4)).

Gorden sign: Pinch the gastrocnemius muscle (Fig. 211 (5)).

Chaddock sign: Draw lines using a bamboo spike or a dull needle along the lateral dorsum of foot (see Fig 211 (3)).

Tuina Manoeuvres

Principal methods: Apply Rolling, Pressing, Kneading, Rubbing with Both Palms, Knocking with the Palm Base, Dotting with the Middle Finger and Straight-rubbing to the back and lower limbs; apply Rolling, Pressing, Kneading, Dredging the Channels, Grasping, Twisting, Rubbing with Both Palms, Rotating and Regulating to the upper limbs; use Pressing, Wiping, Pushing-wiping and Grasping with the Five Fingers on the head.

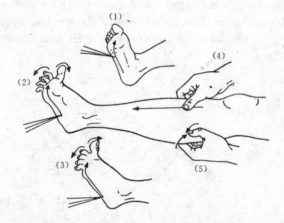

Fig. 211   Examination of the Pathological Plantar Reflex
(1) Bainski's sign (−) (2) Babinski's sign (+)
(3) Chaddock sign (+) (4) Oppenheim sign (+)
(5) Gorden sign (+)

Subordinate methods: Press and knead Tianshu (ST 25), Ganshu (BL 18), Danshu (BL 19), Shenshu (BL 23), Huantiao (GB 30), Yanglingquan (GB 34), Weizhong (BL 40), Fengshi (GB 31), Futu (ST 32), Chengshan (BL 57), Xiyan(Ex−LE)and Jiexi (ST 41) on the back and lower limbs; Chize (LI 5), Quchi (LI 11), Shousanli (LI 10) and Hegu (LI 14) on the upper limbs; Yintang (Ex−HN), Jingming (BL 1), Taiyang (Ex−HN), Fengchi (GB 20), Fengfu (DU 16) and Jianjing (GB 21) on the head and neck.

Perform the operations once a day or every other day.

Case

Ma, female, 53, worker. First visit: May 7th, 1984.

Symptoms: Paralysis and weakness in left limbs, accompanied with aphasia.

Case history: The patient suddenly got the symptoms mentioned-above 3 months ago. Her condition was diagnosed as "cerebral thrombasis". She was given treatment with intravenous drip of glucose and cytidine diphosphate choline, but was not thoroughly relieved.

170

Physical examination: Myodynamic in left limbs with three-graded mypermyotonia; difficulty in flexing and extending the index and middle fingers; positive test in Hoffman's, Babinskin's, Oppenheim Gorden and Chaddock sign); pale purplish tongue with thin and whitish fur; tight pulse. Diagnosis: Hemipleigia due to Qi Deficiency and Blood Stasis.

Cure: After 2 treatments, the left limbs were instantly relaxed and the joints turned to a better condition. After 2 weeks of Tuina therapy, the patient could walk independently with the a stick. With 2 more months of treatments (1 treatment every other day), she was able to walk without stick and muscular tension was higher. 2 years later when she was followed up , it was learnt that she could live on herself.

Gynaecology

1. Dysmenorrhea

Dysmenorrhea refers to severe distending pain in the lower abdomen or lumbar regions before or during menstruation. The patient usually gets pale comlexion, cold sweating on the forehead, cold limbs, nausea, and vomiting along with the menstruation cycle.

Etiology and Pathogenesis

This disease is usually cause by Qi Stagnation and Blood Stasis, or Cold and Dampness, or Qi and Blood Deficiency which bring about disturbance of Qi in movement and Blood in flow in the Chong and Ren Channels and the uterus. It is believed in the modern medicine that such factors as local pathological changes in the genitals, dyspasia of the uterus, stenosis and polyp of the cervix as well as panic, fidgets, debility, affection of Pathogenic Wind and Cold may also lead to the disease.

Clinical Manifestations

Sharp pain occurs in the abdominal or even lumbar regions before or during menstruation, complicated by nausea, vomiting, dizziness and cold limbs in the severe case. The pain disappears automatically after menstruation. The case due to Qi Stagnation and Blood Stasis is often marked by purple menses with blood lumps and deep uneven pulse; the case due to Cold and Dampness marked by pain in abdomen, dark menses as well as whitish and greasy coating and deep tense pulse; the case due to Qi and Blood Deficiency marked by lingering pain in abdomen, relieved with pressure, pale watery menses, as well as lassitude, listlessness, whitish thin coating of the tongue and thread weak pulse.

Tuina Manoeuvres

Principal methods: First, carry out the following manoeuvres on the lower abdomen: Round-rubbing clockwise for 3－5 minutes, Kneading and On-the-point-pressing at Qihai (REN 6) and Guanyuan (REN 4) for 1－2 minutes, and Vibrating for 3－5 minutes. Afterwards, dirigate on the back and lumbar regions along the Bladder Channel by Rolling for 3－5 minutes, Pressing and Kneading at Shenshu (BL 23) and Eight-liaos until the patient perceives a distending and hot sensation on the locale, and Vibrating on the lumbosacral portion for 3－5 minutes.

Subordinate methods: In the case of Qi Stagnation and Blood Stasis, knead Zhangmen (LIV 13) and Qimen (LIV 14), grasp Xuehai (SP 10)and Sanyinjiao (ST 6); in the case of Cold and Dampness, rub the area along the Du Channel on the back and the lumbar region where Shenshu(BL 23) and Mingmen (DU 4) locate horizontally, then press and knead Xuehai (SP 10) and Sanyinjiao (ST 6); in the case of Qi and Blood Deficiency, stroke Zhongwan (REN 12), press Pishu (BL 20), Weishu (BL 21) and Zusanli (ST 36), then run the left portion of the back transversely. In clinical practice, it is commonly performed 5－7 days before menstruation once a day and stopped during menstruation.

Case

Xu, female, 24. First visit: May 6th, 1982.

Symptoms: Distending pain in the lower abdomen before menstruation for more than 2 years.

Case history: She got swelling pain in lower abdomen 3 days before menstruation in Apr. 1980, accompanied with lumps of menses, nausea, cold perspiration or forehead. The pain was relieved when dark menses was discharged and aggravated with emotional depression. No effective result has been achieved with oral administration of Chinese medicine, she came for Tuina therapy.

Physical examination: Suffering complexion with dysphasia; tenderness (+) in the hypogastriam; slight purplish tongue with ecchymosis; uneven pulse.

Diagnosis: Dysmenorrhea due to Qi Stagnation and Blood Stasis.

Cure: After 15 minutes of Tuina manipulation as mentioned-above, pain in low abdomen was instantly relieved. After 2 treatments, the patient only got low-grade pain in lower abdomen. With 3 more treatments, she completely recovered. No recurrence was heard when she was followed up half a year later.

2. Amenorrhea

Amenorrhea refers to no menstruation or discontinued menstruation for more than 3 months in women who are beyond 18 years old.

Etiology and Pathogenesis

Amenorrhea may be caused by various factors: depressed emotions, resulting in Liver Qi Stagnation and Blood Stasis in the Chong and Ren Channels; or attack of exopathic Cold, leading to the generation of Pathogenic Cold and Blood Stasis in the Chong and Ren Channels; or obesity with excessive Phlegm and Dampness, which linger in the Chong Channel and Ren Channels, leading to obstruction of the Bao Channel; or insufficiency of Kidney Qi due to congenital factors or multiparity, which impair the Liver and Kidney, thus leading to blood Deficiency and as a result loss of nutrients in the Chong as well as Ren Channels.

Clinical Manifestations

Amenorrhea due to Qi Stagnation and Blood Stasis: Mainly marked by depression, restlessness, distending pain in the lower abdomen, appearance of ecchymosis on the tongue surface, wiry and uneven pulse.

Amenorrhea due to Phlegm-Dampness: Characterized by a fat figure, tight and depressed feeling in the chest, vomiting, profuse sputum , lassitude in the loins and lower limbs, hot sensation in the palms and soles, greasy tongue coating and slippery pulse.

Amenorrhea due to Liver-Kidney Deficiency: Marked by dizziness, soreness and lassitude of the loins and legs, dysphoria with feverish sensation in the chest, palms and soles, as well as a dim complexion, pale tongue with thin whitish fur, and thread wiry pulse.

Amenorrhea due to Qi-Blood Asthenia: Shown by gradual disappearance of menses, sallow complexion, vertigo, palpatation, shortness of breath, lassitude, anorexia, loose bowels, pale tongue as well as pale lips, and thread weak pulse.

Tuina Manoeuvres

Principal methods: Adopt Round-rubbing, Pressing and Kneading on the lower abdomen; then use Rolling, Pressing and Kneading on the patient's back regions.

Subordinate methods: Press and knead Guanyuan (REN 4) and Qihai(REN 6) on the lower abdomen; Xuehai (SP 10), Sanyinjiao (ST 6) and Zusanli (ST 36) on the lower limbs; Ganshu (BL 18), Pishu(BL 20), Weishu (BL 21) and Shenshu (BL 23) on the back.

In addition to the Tuina methods mentioned-above, rub the sacral region in a straight line, then press and knead Eight-liaoss, in the case of Qi Stagnation and Blood Stasis; rub the left portion of the back and lumbosacral regions, and press and knead Zhongwan (REN 12), Zusanli(ST 36) in the case of Phlegm and Dampness; rub along the line where locate Shenshu (BL 23) and Mingmen (DU 4)in the case of Liver and Kidney Deficiency; rub the Du Channel on the back and the left side of the back, then pinch the muscles along the spine, in the case of Qi and Blood Deficiency, until the patient perceives a local deepening, penetrating and burning sensation.

Carry out the dirigation once a day or every other day for 12 times in succession as a therapeutic course.

3. Acute Mastitis

Acute mastitis often occurs during the woman's breast feeding period in her first child birth.

Etiology and Pathogenesis

Acute Mastitis may be caused by cracked, deformed or crater nip-

174

ples during lactation; or caused by hyperlactation which results in retention of milk and thus the obstruction of the Collaterals in charge of milk secretion; or by emotional stimulation and improper diet, which lead to incoordination of the Liver and the Spleen, Qi Stagnation and Blood Stasis, obstruction of the Channels and Collaterals, and consequently supportive mammary masses.

Clinical Manifestations

The disease is marked by distension, swelling, perceivable mass and para-eccrisis of milk in the affected breast, accompanied by chill, fever, headache, poor appetite, general aching and malaise. At the armpit of the diseased side, swelling is perceived and tends to be enlarging. At the later stage, the centre of the swelling has ulceration and may not heal until the pus has been completely excreted.

Tuina Manoeuvres

Principal methods: First, Rub and knead the area around the breast with the fingers (Fig. 212); secondly, push and rub from the base of the breast to its nipple with the palm (see Fig. 213); thirdly, knead and rub the abdominal regions; finally, manipulate by Pressing, Grasping and Kneading on the neck and upper limbs, Rolling, Pressing and Kneading on the back along the Bladder Channel.

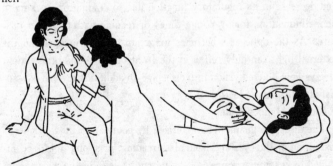

Fig. 212 Rubbing-kneading around the Breast with the Fingers

Fig. 213 Pushing-rubbing from the Mammary Base to the Nipple

175

Subordinate methods: Press and knead Ganshu (BL 18), Pishu (BL 20), Weishu (BL 21), Fengchi (GB 20), Jianjing (GB 21), Shaoze (SI 1), Hegu (LI 4), Ganshu (BL 19), Pishu (BL 20) and Weishu (BL 21).

It is recommended that Tuina therapy be carried out at the initial stage of acute mastitis before the appearance of infection. The manipulations should be performed mildly, softly, briskly, and dexterously first in the vicinity of the swollen mass, then to its center, once every day.

Five Sense Organs

1. Myopia

Myopia refers to the morbid condition of the eye, caused by ametropia, occurring mostly in youths and teenagers. Clinically, it is classified into two types: pseudomyopia and genuine myopia. The former responds better to Tuina practice than the later.

Etiology and Pathogenesis

The disease is mainly caused by overstrain of the ciliary muscle and decrease in its regulatory function due to reading or working in poor illumination for over long time, or reading with improper posture. As the optic axis becomes longer in genuine myopia and the external light can only reflex in the front of the retina, the patient always gets blurred vision in far-seeing. In addition, myopia is associated with genetic factors.

Clinical Manifestations

The disease is mainly characterized by poor far-seeing, dizziness, distention of the eyes and head after reading for a long time, accompanied by insomnia, amnesia, aching and malaise of the waist. Furthermore, there occurs evident soreness, distention or Heat sensation at the points like Jingming (BL 1) and Sibai (ST 2) when pressed. The disease can be easily diagnosed through the visual method, funduscopy and optomery.

Tuina Manoeuvres

Principal methods: Manipulate by Pushing the Forehead Divergently, Pinching the Eyebrows, Wiping, Pressing-kneading the Orbits (Fig. 214), Pressing-kneading the Superciliary Arches (Fig. 215), Grasping the Neck and Vibrating on Jingming (BL 1).

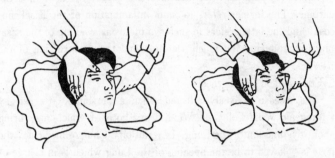

Fig. 214 Pressing-kneading   Fig. 215 Pressing-kneading
the Orbits   the Superciliary Arches

Subordinate methods: Press and knead Jingming (BL 1), Yintang (Ex−HN), Yuyao (Ex−HN), Sibai (ST 2), Fengchi (GB 20), Ganshu (BL 18) and Hegu (LI 4).

Treat the disease once a day.

Case

Liu, male, 18. First visit: Sep. 23rd, 1990.

Symptoms: Poor farseeing for 3 months.

Case history: Three months ago, the patient began to suffer from blurred vision in far-seeing, hypopsia (diminution of vision) and blepsopathia, accompanied by dizziness, distension of the head, dryness and foreign body sensation in the eyes. He once accepted treatment in another hospital by oral administration of Chinese medicine and acupuncture, but failed to have any help.

Physical examination: Weary complexion; visual acuity: 4. 8 in the left eye and 4. 7 in the right eye; tenderness (+) at Jingming (BL 1) and Yuyao (Ex−HN); pink tongue and deep, thread and wiry pulse.

Diagnosis: Myopia (Pseudomyopia).

Cure: After 1 Tuina treatment (about 10 minutes), the patient felt relaxed and comfortable in his eyes. 6 times later, his morbid state changed a lot. Two more weeks of Tuna therapy found his symptoms and signs basically cleared up.

2. Rhinitis

Clinically, Rhinitis is divided into two types: the acute and the chronic. The former refers to acute inflammation of the nasal mucosa, and the latter refers to such symptoms as swelling of the nasal mucosa producing too much secretion and thus obstruction of the nasal cavity.

Etiology and Pathogenesis

The disease is easily affected when a person is attacked by Pathogenic Wind-Cold and Wind-Heat, both of which may bring about dysfunction of the Lung. In traditional Chinese medicine, the nose is believed to be the opening of the Lung which is in charge of respiration and skin of the human body surface. When the Lung is attacked by exogenous factors, there will be lingering of noxious factors in the nasal passage, thus the disease.

Clinical Manifestations

Acute Rhinitis: Marked mainly by swelling of the nasal mucosa, stuffy nose, watery nasal discharge, complicated by headache, pyrexia, aversion to wind, reddened tongue with thin whitish fur, floating and rapid pulse.

Chronic Rhinitis: Manifested as diffuse hyperemia, thickening or atrophy of the nasal mucosa, excessive nasal secretion, turbid nasal discharge, complicated by rhinophonia, dryness of the nasal mucosa, broadening of the nasal cavity and hyposphresia. The tongue is usually red, the fur yellowish and the pulse rapid.

Tuina Manoeuvres

Principal methods: Use Rubbing-Kneading on either side of the nose, Pressing-kneading at various points of the face, Grasping on the neck and at Jianjing (GB 21).

Subordinate methods: Press and knead Yingxiang (LI 20), Yintang (Ex—HN), Fengchi (GB 20), Feishu (BL 13) and Hegu (LI

178

4).

In addition to the routine manoeuvres mentioned-above, knead Fengmen (BL 12), rub the Bladder Channel on the back until the patient perceives a local burning sensation in Wind-Cold Syndrome; knead Dazhui (DU 14) and Quchi (LI 11) and rub the Bladder Channel on the back until there appears slight redness on the locale in Wind-Heat Syndrome.

The treatment should be given once a day or once 2 days.

Case

Wang, male, 32. First visit: Dec. 18th, 1990.

Symptoms: Alternative nasal obstruction and turbid nasal discharge for more than 3 months.

Case history: The patient was affected by cold in September, 1990. Thereafter, he suffered from stuffy nose, sneezing, abundant watery nasal discharge, together with pyrexia (T 37.5 C), as well as sore-throat. A week later, all the symptoms and signs were basically assuaged. However, he was broken down with alternative nasal obstruction, aggravated at night, turbid nasal discharge, accompanied by low-grade pain and distension in the head. He once accepted treatment by Chinese and western medicines in another hospital, but failed to have obvious effects. So he came for Tuina treatment.

Physical examination: Hyperemia of the nasal mucosa, hypertrophic conchae, flushed nose, copious yellowish snivel, in combination with hyposmia, pale complexion, lassitude, listlessness,, pale tongue with thin yellowish fur and deep thread pulse.

Diagnosis: Chronic Rhinitis.

Cure: After 1 treatment (10 minutes or so), the patient felt his systoms relieved a lot. Six times more in succession, he was basically recovered. To obtain better results, he was treated by manipulation once 2 days for an extra month and all the symptoms and signs were gone. Half a year later, we made follow-ups and no recurrence of the disease was found.

3. Toothache

Toothache, in traditional Chinese medicine, is subcategorized into

Excess Syndrome and Deficiency Syndrome. The former is mostly caused by Stomach Fire and the latter by Kidney Deficiency.

Etiology and Pathogenesis

The onset of the disease is presupposed mostly by such factors as accumulation of Heat in the Stomach, in combination with Pathogenic Wind and Heat, or by Kidney Deficiency producing Deficiency of Fire, which lead to the pathological changes in the gum. Furthermore, dental caries out of putrefaction of the gum may also lead toothache.

Clinical Manifestations

Toothache due to Stomach Fire: Marked by pain in the affected teeth, aggravated by stimuli such as cold, hot, sour, sweet factors, accompanied by redness, swelling and pus discharge in the gum, foul breath, thirst, constipation, deep colored urine, reddened tongue with thick yellowish coating and rapid pulse.

Toothache of Kidney Deficiency: Manifested with slackened teeth, vague pain in the diseased area, aggravated in chewing or after the noon, redness in the affected gum, dry throat, reddened tongue with little coating and thread rapid pulse.

Toothache due to caries occurs when the gum is stimulated by cold or heat or when the dental cavity is stuffed with food.

Tuina Manoeuvres

Principal methods: Treat the disease by Pressing with the Thumb and Kneading with the Finger.

Subordinate methods: Press and knead with a finger Jiache (ST 6), Xiaguan (ST 7), Hegu (LI 4) and Yatong (MA) (locating at the spot 1 cun from the transverse crease of the palm between the 3rd and 4th metacarpal bones).

In addition, knead Taichong (LIV 3) in its severe case of the disease; knead Taixi (KID 9) in the case of Deficiency of Fire; press and knead Neiting (ST 44) and Fengchi (GB 20) in the case of Pathogenic Wind and Heat.

The treatment is better to be given once a day.

Notes

Pay attention to oral hygiene. Brush teeth before sleep. Avoid

180

stimulating the teeth by cold or heat. Try to prevent dental caries and go to see a doctor as long as the onset of cariogenesis begins.

推拿疗法

编　　著　王道全

译　　者　闫梦辉

　　　　　张　帆

责任编辑　李　宇

*

山东科学技术出版社出版

济南市玉函路 16 号　邮政编码　250002

山东德州新华印刷厂印刷

中国国际图书贸易总公司发行

中国北京车公庄西路 35 号

北京邮政信箱第 399 号　邮政编码　100044

*

1996 年（大 32 开）　1 版 1 次

ISBN 7－5331－1839－1

R・532

07200

14－E－3019P